Fast Facts

D0920569

Rheumatoid Arthritis

Second edition

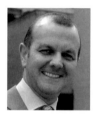

John D Isaacs PhD FRCP
Professor of Clinical Rheumatology and Director
Wilson Horne Immunotherapy Centre
Newcastle University
Consultant Rheumatologist, Freeman Hospital
Newcastle-upon-Tyne, UK

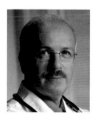

Larry W Moreland MD
Chief of Rheumatology
Division of Rheumatology and Clinical Immunology
University of Pittsburgh
USA

Declaration of Independence
This book is as balanced and as practical as we can make it.
Ideas for improvement are always welcome: feedback@fastfacts.com

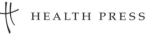 HEALTH PRESS

Fast Facts: Rheumatoid Arthritis
First published 2002
Second edition May 2011

Text © 2011 John D Isaacs, Larry W Moreland
© 2011 in this edition Health Press Limited
Health Press Limited, Elizabeth House, Queen Street, Abingdon,
Oxford OX14 3LN, UK
Tel: +44 (0)1235 523233
Fax: +44 (0)1235 523238

Book orders can be placed by telephone or via the website.
For regional distributors or to order via the website, please go to:
www.fastfacts.com
For telephone orders, please call +44 (0)1752 202301 (UK, Europe and Asia–
Pacific), 1 800 247 6553 (USA, toll free) or +1 419 281 1802 (Americas).

Fast Facts is a trademark of Health Press Limited.

A CIP record for this title is available from the British Library.

ISBN 978-1-905832-91-0

Isaacs JD (John)
Fast Facts: Rheumatoid Arthritis/
John D Isaacs, Larry W Moreland

Medical illustrations by Dee McLean, London, UK.
Typesetting and page layout by Zed, Oxford, UK.
Printed in China with Xpedient Print Services.

Introduction

Rheumatoid arthritis (RA) is the commonest inflammatory joint disease, affecting approximately 1% of adults in the developed world. Here, we provide an easy-to-read and up-to-date overview of how RA is thought to develop, how it is diagnosed and monitored, and how it is treated, incorporating the major advances in these areas that have taken place since the first edition.

The pathogenesis of RA is starting to become unraveled and, more than in any other disease, this has led to powerful targeted treatments. Specifically, nine targeted biological therapies have, at the time of press, received approval by regulatory agencies. These target inflammatory mediators and the cells that coordinate the dysregulated immune and inflammatory responses that characterize RA. They are discussed in the closing chapters of the book, along with our thoughts on future directions of investigation and management. We also cover the new classification criteria for RA, and a new autoantibody class, anti-citrullinated peptide antibody (ACPA), is discussed in the context of its use for diagnosing RA.

Synovium

The synovial membrane lines the non-weight-bearing aspects of the synovial cavity and is divided into the lining layer or intima and sublining layer or subintima. It is the target tissue of the dysregulated inflammation and immunity that characterizes rheumatoid arthritis (RA) (Figure 1.1). The synovial membrane intima is just one or two cell layers thick and contains two major cell types: type A synoviocytes, which bear macrophage markers, and type B synoviocytes, which have fibroblastic characteristics. The intima lacks the typical features of an epithelium and does not possess a basement membrane or tight intercellular contacts between synoviocytes. The matrix of the intima is rich in proteoglycans and glycosaminoglycans, in particular hyaluronic acid.

The subintima is a loose vascular connective tissue stroma containing blood vessels, lymphatics and nerve endings within a

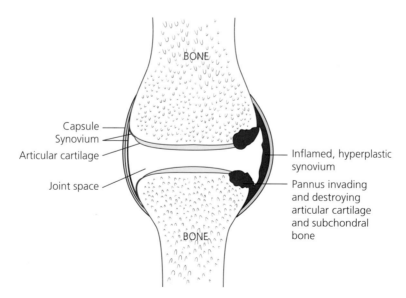

Figure 1.1 Normal joint anatomy (left side of figure) and RA pathology (right).

matrix comprising varying proportions of lipid, collagen fibrils and more organized fibrous tissue.

Synovial fluid

The synovial membrane secretes lubricating and nourishing synovial fluid, a viscous fluid containing a high concentration of hyaluronic acid. Other constituents include nutrients and solutes that diffuse from the blood vessels in the subintima. The precise physiology of synovial fluid production is unknown, but exchange of fluid between the circulation and the joint space is governed by a balance of hydrostatic, osmotic and convective forces. As well as providing an osmotic force within the synovial cavity, hyaluronic acid contributes to the lubricating properties of synovial fluid although other constituents are also important.

Articular cartilage

Articular cartilage comprises chondrocytes embedded in a hydrated matrix composed of collagen, proteoglycans and other matrix proteins. It is an avascular structure lacking lymphatics, and the synovial fluid is critical for providing nutrients to this tissue. Water makes up approximately 70% of normal cartilage by weight, whereas chondrocytes occupy only 5–10% by volume. Because of their low density, chondrocytes do not come into contact with one another directly but possess cellular processes which abut the matrix. These cells are critical to the integrity of articular cartilage because they synthesize collagen, proteoglycans and also other components such as fibronectin. Each cell is surrounded by a zone of secreted proteoglycans and a basket-like mantle of fibrillar collagen, but the highest collagen content occurs in the more distal intercellular matrix.

Collagens are fibrillar proteins that, together with proteoglycans, account for the biomechanical properties of articular cartilage. There are 14 different types of collagen, divided into three major groups. The predominant collagen in articular cartilage is type II, constituting approximately 90% in the adult, with types IX and XI contributing most of the remainder. All collagens are based on a triple helical structure (Figure 1.2), and the differences between collagens relate to

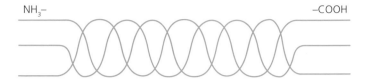

Figure 1.2 The triple helix gives collagen tensile strength.

the length of the triple helix, the presence of non-collagenous units within the molecule that impart extra flexibility, or the addition of non-collagenous side-chains such as carbohydrates. The triple helical structure of collagens accounts for their tensile strength. Collagen biosynthetic and degradative pathways are quite well characterized.

Proteoglycans are large negatively charged macromolecules comprising a polypeptide core with glycosaminoglycan side-chains. The largest family of proteoglycans in articular cartilage is the aggrecans, which contain abundant chondroitin sulfate and keratan sulfate side-chains. They are complexed with hyaluronic acid and so-called link protein. Their main function relates to their anionic and water-trapping properties, which provide deformability and compressibility. The ratio of collagen to aggrecan is high in the superficial layers of articular cartilage and drops progressively toward the subchondral bone. Thus, the surface layers have high tensile strength and resilience whereas the lower layers have higher deformability and compressibility. During load-bearing, water and solutes are squeezed out of aggrecan, which increases the relative proteoglycan concentration, providing an osmotic drive to rehydration once the load is removed.

Breakdown of collagen and the surrounding matrix is mediated by enzymes such as collagenase, gelatinase, stromelysin and aggrecanase, which are zinc-dependent metalloproteinases. In turn, these enzymes are controlled by tissue inhibitors of metalloproteinases (TIMPs). Thus, tissue homeostasis is maintained by carefully balanced synthetic and catabolic pathways. Cartilage thinning and breakdown (chondrolysis) can be precipitated by either excessive loading or disuse. In osteoarthritis, genetic factors also contribute to loss of cartilage integrity (see *Fast Facts: Osteoarthritis*). In disease states such as RA, pro-inflammatory cytokines such as interleukin-1 (IL-1), and tumor necrosis factor (TNF) reduce synthesis and increase catabolism of articular cartilage, leading to rapid breakdown. In contrast, growth factors such as transforming growth factor β (TGFβ) and insulin-like growth factor-1 (IGF-1) stimulate synthesis of cartilage components.

Subchondral bone

The basal layer of articular cartilage is calcified and is attached directly to subchondral bone, which has a similar structure. Collagen I comprises most of the collagen present in bone, however, and is calcified with hydroxyapatite. This provides bone with both tensile and compressive strength. The remaining bone matrix is made up of proteoglycans, glycoproteins, glycosaminoglycans such as hyaluronic acid, and proteins such as osteocalcin; as in articular cartilage, these are incorporated into macromolecular complexes. Glycoproteins such as osteopontin, osteonectin and bone sialoproteins function as anchoring molecules, bridging matrix constituents such as collagen to bone cells. Bone also contains important growth factors such as IGF-1 and 2, and the bone morphogenetic proteins (BMPs) which are members of the TGFβ superfamily.

Formation and destruction. Bone contains two major cell types: osteoblasts and osteoclasts. Mesenchymal osteoblasts are critical for the synthesis of collagen and bone matrix (osteoid). Conversely, osteoclasts – multinucleate cells of macrophage lineage – break down bone via a combination of lysosomal enzymes and low pH. Bone is constantly remodeled to fulfill two major functions.
- To optimize load-bearing capacity, bone is remodeled according to compressive forces acting upon it.
- Bone remodeling also plays an important role in metabolic homeostasis, particularly of calcium and magnesium.

Therefore, in addition to mechanical forces, stimuli to bone formation and breakdown include circulating hormones and vitamins, such as parathyroid hormone, thyroid hormone, vitamin D, calcitonin and sex hormones (Figure 1.3).

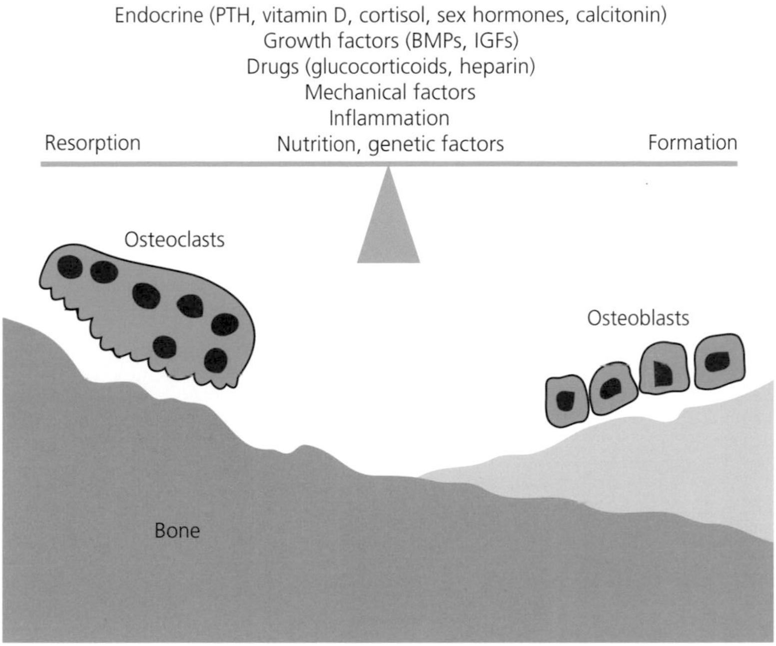

Endocrine (PTH, vitamin D, cortisol, sex hormones, calcitonin)
Growth factors (BMPs, IGFs)
Drugs (glucocorticoids, heparin)
Mechanical factors
Inflammation
Resorption | Nutrition, genetic factors | Formation

Osteoclasts

Osteoblasts

Bone

Figure 1.3 The balance between bone synthesis and breakdown represents the integration of several influences. BMP, bone morphogenetic protein; IGF, insulin-like growth factor; PTH, parathyroid hormone.

In young adults, bone formation and destruction are carefully balanced to maintain overall bone mass. In the elderly, however, and particularly in postmenopausal women, breakdown may exceed synthesis, leading to osteoporosis (see *Fast Facts: Osteoporosis*). Resorption is also accelerated by drugs such as corticosteroids, and by inflammation. Bone density measurements using dual emission X-ray absorptiometry (DEXA), ultrasound or quantitative CT (qCT) provide surrogate measures of bone strength and fracture risk.

Key points – the normal joint

- The joint is a complex organ composed of a number of specialized tissues.
- Dysregulation within any one of the tissues within the joint may precipitate specific pathologies, such as osteoarthritis or osteoporosis. In rheumatoid arthritis, the primary pathological target is the synovial membrane.

Key references

Compston JE, Rosen CJ. *Fast Facts: Osteoporosis*, 6th edn. Oxford: Health Press, 2009.

Conaghan P, Sharma L. *Fast Facts: Osteoarthritis*. Oxford: Health Press, 2009.

Firestein G, Budd RC, Harris ED et al., eds. *Kelley's Textbook of Rheumatology*, 8th edn. Philadelphia: Saunders, 2008.

Hochberg MC, Silman AJ, Smolen JS et al., eds. *Rheumatology*, 4th edn. St Louis: Mosby, 2007.

Isenberg D, Maddison P, Woo P et al., eds. *Oxford Textbook of Rheumatology*, 3rd edn. New York: Oxford University Press, 2004.

Koopman WJ, Moreland LW, eds. *Arthritis and Allied Conditions*. Philadelphia: Lippincott Williams & Wilkins, 2005.

As with many common diseases, rheumatoid arthritis (RA) represents a balance between nature and nurture, in which environmental factors act upon a genetically predisposed host. In the past few years great advances have been made in dissecting the gene–environment interactions that predispose to RA.

Genetic factors

Family studies and twin studies indicate that there is a genetic susceptibility to RA, which is higher in families with more severe disease. Genetic predisposition is estimated to contribute between a half and two-thirds to RA susceptibility. Unlike classic Mendelian diseases such as cystic fibrosis or sickle cell disease, RA is a polygenic and genetically heterogeneous disease. Thus, a number of different genes predispose to RA, and these may differ from patient to patient (Figure 2.1). Essentially, various combinations of polymorphisms in a selection of different genes (genotype) predispose to the clinical picture (phenotype) that is recognized as RA. Additionally, some genes may influence severity rather than occurrence of RA.

Until recently, the major histocompatibility complex (MHC) was the only genetic region that had been consistently linked to RA. This is a large genetic region on the short arm of chromosome 6 that encompasses a variety of genes and contributes approximately one-third of the genetic susceptibility to RA. A large part of the MHC comprises the human leukocyte antigen (HLA) genes. These encode an individual's tissue type and include class I (HLA-A, HLA-B, HLA-C) and class II (HLA-DR, HLA-DQ, HLA-DP) genes. The encoded proteins are critical in determining the manner by which an individual's immune system recognizes and responds to provocative stimuli, and the MHC also contains many other genes related to immune function. The strongest genetic link to RA is the class II HLA region and, in particular, *HLA-DRB1*. HLA-DR molecules comprise an invariant alpha chain (encoded by *HLA-DRA*) and a highly

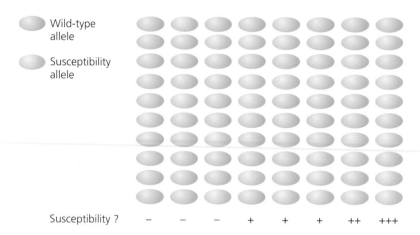

Figure 2.1 Genetics of a complex disease such as rheumatoid arthritis (RA). Each vertical line represents an individual, for whom ten potential susceptibility genes are indicated (there are many more than this). Each gene possesses a 'wild-type' (green) and a 'susceptibility' (yellow) allele. For the current argument, a predisposition to RA requires the inheritance of four or more susceptibility alleles. Only one allele is shown for each gene, and it is assumed that the alternative allele is wild type in every case. Some individuals inherit none or fewer than four susceptibility alleles and are not prone to develop RA. Others inherit four or more, resulting in a variable predisposition. Note that predisposition can involve completely different groups of genes, accounting for the phenotypic heterogeneity of RA. In RA, the shared epitope provides the main genetic risk factor.

polymorphic beta chain (encoded by *HLA-DRB1*), and constitute a platform upon which antigenic peptides are presented to and seen by the immune system. Particular HLA-DRB1 molecules are more common in individuals with RA, and these share a sequence in a part of the molecule that influences the peptides that are bound and therefore viewed by the immune system (Figure 2.2). This core amino acid sequence is termed the 'shared epitope'. The shared epitope influences both the incidence and the severity of RA, and individuals who inherit two shared epitope-encoding *HLA-DRB1* alleles suffer particularly aggressive disease.

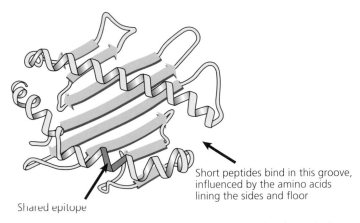

Short peptides bind in this groove, influenced by the amino acids lining the sides and floor

Shared epitope

Figure 2.2 A human leukocyte antigen (HLA)-DR molecule, with the approximate location of the shared epitope indicated.

It has been hypothesized that the shared epitope specifically binds an autoantigen-derived peptide with high affinity, thereby predisposing to an autoimmune arthritis. Although the autoantigen in RA has not been definitively identified, a number have been proposed (see Chapter 3) and, in most cases, specific peptides derived from these proteins can bind to HLA-DR molecules containing the shared epitope.

There are other potential explanations for this genetic association, however. For example, HLA type also biases the repertoire of T cells generated in the thymus, and the shared epitope could, by chance, select T cells with a particular affinity for joint antigens. In this context, non-inherited maternal HLA molecules may also influence RA susceptibility. The shared epitope itself could also become an autoantigen. Certain viruses and bacteria contain an identical peptide sequence within one or other of their proteins. An immune response against the microbe could then trigger an autoimmune response against HLA-DR-expressing cells, a process termed 'molecular mimicry'.

Non-MHC genes. Genome-wide association studies (GWAS) have revolutionized our understanding of complex diseases such as RA. The human genome sequencing project highlighted the abundance of single nucleotide polymorphisms (SNPs) in human DNA. These are single base-pair differences in DNA sequence between different individuals, which do not usually change the function of the gene. The development of high-throughput genotyping technologies has enabled large-scale GWAS in which hundreds of thousands of SNPs that span the entire genome are rapidly compared in patients with a particular disease and matched controls. SNPs that appear more commonly in individuals with the disease in question should lie within or close to genes that are associated with the disease. The Wellcome Trust Case Control Consortium published the first GWAS of RA and, with subsequent studies, has identified and confirmed a number of genes associated with the disease. These include genes encoding proteins such as protein tyrosine phosphatase-22 (PTPN22), an important regulator of lymphocyte activation, cytotoxic T-lymphocyte-associated protein 4 (CTLA-4), a downregulator of T cell activation, and STAT4, a signaling molecule downstream of the interleukin (IL)-12/IL-23 receptor. Table 2.1 lists genetic loci that have been reproducibly linked to RA in populations of European descent. It has been estimated that approximately 35% of the genetic risk for RA has now been established, most of which is attributable to the MHC. Consequently, many minor genetic influences await identification, including more recent concepts such as gene copy number variants.

TABLE 2.1

Confirmed non-HLA genetic associations with rheumatoid arthritis

PTPN22	PRKCQ
STAT4	CD40
TRAF1/C5	MMEL1/TNFRSF14
TNFAIP3/OLIG3	AFF3
IL2RB	IL2–IL21
KIF5A/PIP4K2C	CTLA-4

For more information on the genes listed, go to www.ncbi.nlm.nih.gov/gene. HLA, human leukocyte antigen.

Smoking

A seminal study has irrefutably linked smoking to the etiology of RA in patients carrying a predisposing genotype. A healthy individual carrying two copies of the shared epitope (one on each chromosome 6, see pages 14–15) has an odds ratio (OR) of developing anti-citrullinated peptide antibody (ACPA)-positive RA that is about five times that of someone who is shared-epitope negative. If the individual smokes, the OR increases to approximately 23 times. *PTPN22* also contributes to RA risk in this model, which clearly demonstrates the influence of smoking on RA development (Figure 2.3). Smoking appears to interact

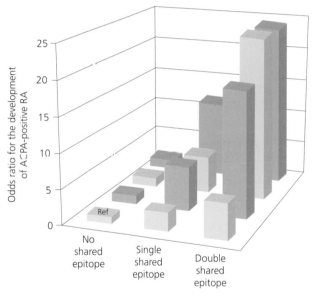

■ Any *PTPN22* R620W, smoking
◻ No *PTPN22* R620W, smoking
■ Any *PTPN22* R620W, no smoking
◻ No *PTPN22* R620W, no smoking

Figure 2.3 The interaction of the shared epitope, smoking and *PTPN22* genotype on the risk of developing rheumatoid arthritis (RA). *PTPN22* R620W is the *PTPN22* polymorphism associated with increased risk of RA. Adapted with permission from Kallberg et al. 2007. ACPA, anti-citrullinated peptide antibody; ref, reference.

with the shared epitope, leading to the production of ACPA, perhaps via the citrullination of proteins in the lung, thereby increasing their immunogenicity. (Citrullination is the post-translational modification of an arginine to form citrulline [see page 61].) Other airborne exposures, for example to silica dust and coal dust, have also been associated with the development of RA. The shared epitope and *PTPN22* appear to be associated only with ACPA-positive RA, and seronegative disease appears to have a distinct, and much less well defined, etiology.

'Pre-RA'

A number of studies over the past 10 years have indicated that the process that culminates in RA may start up to 15 years before signs and symptoms appear. For example, autoantibodies (rheumatoid factor [RF] and ACPA) first appear in blood 10–15 years before clinical onset, suggesting that immune tolerance breaks down around that time. Similarly, inflammatory markers, cytokines and chemokines start to rise or appear in blood around 5 years before symptoms are evident. Whether all individuals who develop autoantibodies will ultimately develop RA is currently uncertain, but there may be important additional environmental triggers for disease onset.

Infectious triggers

Infectious agents can be associated with arthritic illness in both humans and in animals. For example, parvovirus B19 causes a transient illness with features of RA in man, and Lyme disease, a chronic infection by a tick-transmitted spirochete, has chronic joint manifestations. Lentiviruses can cause arthritis in mammals, and HIV may precipitate an arthritic illness in man. Reactive arthritis provides an obvious example of self-limiting arthritis triggered by a variety of bacterial infections. In animals, adjuvant arthritis is triggered by immunization with extracts of mycobacteria. Despite these examples, no consistent association has been found between RA and any infectious agent, and the disease does not occur in clusters or demonstrate seasonal variation. Thus, any infectious trigger may be ubiquitous in different populations, and have a high infectivity.

Epstein–Barr virus (EBV) has been implicated in some studies, and certain EBV proteins provide shared-epitope-binding peptides as well as a sequence that mimics the shared epitope. The absence of an infectious agent in arthritic tissue does not exclude a potential etiologic role, because a transient infection could trigger a chronic inflammatory process. It is also possible that RA is the consequence of a chronic infection with an as yet unidentified organism.

Hormonal factors

RA is more common in women than in men, suggesting a possible effect of sex hormones on susceptibility. Furthermore, RA generally improves during pregnancy and may flare in the puerperium. The age-specific incidence equalizes after the female menopause. Additionally, a number of epidemiological studies have reported a fall in the incidence of RA in women over the past 20–30 years. While the evidence is only suggestive, this has been attributed to a possible protective effect of estrogens in the oral contraceptive pill. Hormone replacement therapy has also been suggested as protective in some but not all studies.

Stress and trauma have been reported to trigger RA in some individuals, which may be related to putative defects in hypothalamic–pituitary–adrenal axis regulation (Chapter 3).

Diet

Many patients report that certain foods seem to trigger episodes of arthritis. There is little consistency between patients, however, and controlled trials of dietary intervention have failed to implicate particular classes of foodstuff. These would only provide positive results, however, if patients shared a common dietary trigger whereas individuals generally identify different triggers. Starvation improves RA symptoms, and a few studies have incriminated a high-protein diet as an arthritogenic trigger. Obesity is also associated with RA in a few epidemiological studies, as is caffeine consumption. A 'Mediterranean' diet, and a diet rich in antioxidants may be protective. Others have reported omega-3 polyunsaturated fatty acids, as found in fish oils, to be potentially therapeutic, possibly via an effect on prostaglandin synthesis. Evening primrose oil could have similar anti-inflammatory effects. Recently, alcohol consumption has been reported to protect against RA development. These effects are generally weak and the study results inconsistent, but research continues in the area of diet and arthritis.

A unifying model

It is now possible to construct a simple unifying model for seropositive RA (Figure 2.4). In brief, a susceptible individual inherits a collection of predisposing alleles, which might include a shared-epitope-encoding *HLA-DRB1* allele and an RA-associated *PTPN22* allele. It is notable that many of the genes associated with seropositive RA encode proteins that affect immune cell function and are also associated with other autoimmune diseases. For example, both PTPN22 and CTLA-4 influence T cell activation, and are also associated with type 1 diabetes. The immune effects of these genes may be relevant either in the tissues, by prolonging immune responses, or potentially in the thymus by influencing positive and negative selection of T cells. It now

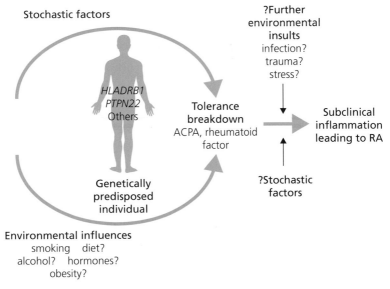

Figure 2.4 A unifying model of rheumatoid arthritis (RA) etiology (see text for details). ACPA, anti-citrullinated peptide antibody.

appears that smoking triggers the formation of ACPA in genetically predisposed individuals, and that this occurs some years before disease onset. Subsequently, a further environmental event may trigger subclinical inflammation, eventually culminating in clinical disease. The precise role of the shared epitope is unclear, but some citrullinated peptides bind more strongly to shared epitope alleles than their non-citrullinated counterparts. In this context, it is also interesting that the gene encoding peptidyl arginine deiminase-4 (PADI-4), an enzyme that catalyzes citrullination, is associated with RA in some ethnic groups.

Stochastic factors

Identical twins (who inherit identical genetic material and usually share the same environment) may nonetheless be discordant for RA. This suggests that random, or stochastic, events are also required for disease expression. Possibilities include somatic genetic events such as T or B cell receptor gene rearrangements, or perhaps epigenetic events. These concepts are difficult to prove and lie outside the scope of this text. Nonetheless they should probably be incorporated into models designed to explain the etiology of RA.

Key points – etiology

- Genetic and environmental factors both play a role in the etiology of RA. A number of genetic associations with RA have now been identified.
- Smoking is an important environmental trigger that, in shared-epitope-positive individuals, stimulates the production of anti-citrullinated peptide antibodies (ACPAs).
- Autoantibodies appear up to 15 years before clinical disease is manifest, suggesting a further influence of additional environmental triggers at a later time point.
- Subclinical inflammation starts to manifest approximately 5 years before disease onset.

Key references

Aggarwal R, Liao K, Nair R et al. Anti-citrullinated peptide antibody assays and their role in the diagnosis of rheumatoid arthritis. *Arthritis Rheum* 2009;61:1472–83.

Anon. Genome-wide association study of 14,000 cases of seven common diseases and 3,000 shared controls. *Nature* 2007;447:661–78.

Kallberg H, Padyukov L, Plenge RM et al. Gene-gene and gene-environment interactions involving HLA-DRB1, PTPN22, and smoking in two subsets of rheumatoid arthritis. *Am J Hum Genet* 2007;80:867–75.

Karlson EW, Chibnik LB, Tworoger SS et al. Biomarkers of inflammation and development of rheumatoid arthritis in women from two prospective cohort studies. *Arthritis Rheum* 2009;60:641–52.

Klareskog L, Catrina AI, Paget S. Rheumatoid arthritis. *Lancet* 2009;373:659–72.

Mahdi H, Fisher BA, Kallberg H, et al. Specific interaction between genotype, smoking and autoimmunity to citrullinated alpha-enolase in the etiology of rheumatoid arthritis. *Nat Genet* 2009;41:1319–24.

Nielen MM, van Schaardenburg D, Reesink HW et al. Specific autoantibodies precede the symptoms of rheumatoid arthritis: a study of serial measurements in blood donors. *Arthritis Rheum* 2004;50:380–6.

Wegner N, Lundberg K, Kinloch A et al. Autoimmunity to specific citrullinated proteins gives the first clues to the etiology of rheumatoid arthritis. *Immunol Rev* 2010;233:34–54.

The fundamental pathology in rheumatoid arthritis (RA) is destruction of articular cartilage and subchondral bone by ectopic and hyperplastic synovium. A variety of models have been proposed to account for this outcome, each with some experimental support.

Rheumatoid synovitis

The synovial membrane in RA becomes hyperplastic and, on direct visualization, may be thrown into villous-like folds (Figure 3.1). Both the lining layer and the sublining demonstrate characteristic changes on microscopy (Figure 3.2). The lining demonstrates an increased number of both type A and type B synoviocytes, and increases from the normal two to three cell layers up to ten cell layers in thickness (Figure 3.3). The sublining becomes infiltrated with immune and inflammatory cells, particularly macrophages, B and T lymphocytes, plasma cells and dendritic cells. Lymphoid follicles may be present, resembling germinal centers of lymph nodes. Neovascularization is dramatic and an essential feature of the hyperplastic sublining layer.

As the disease progresses, the nature of the synovium changes. The synoviocytes ignore their normal tissue boundaries and migrate onto

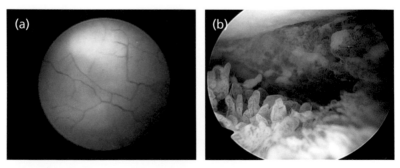

Figure 3.1. Macrosopic appearance of normal (a) and inflamed (b) synovium. Normal synovium is translucent, revealing underlying blood vessels; the inflamed synovium shows villus formation, increased vascularity and fibrin deposition. Images courtesy of Dr R. Reece and Dr J. Canete.

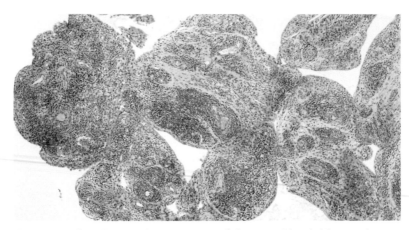

Figure 3.2 The microscopic appearance of rheumatoid arthritis synovium. The normally thin and delicate synovial membrane is invaded by inflammatory cells with plentiful lymphoid aggregates. There is abundant neovascularization and areas of tissue edema. H&E staining, original magnification x 4. Image courtesy of Dr J. Canete.

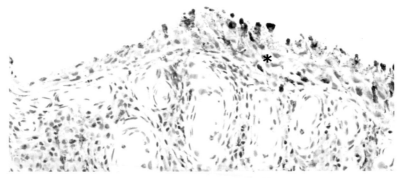

Figure 3.3 Detail of rheumatoid arthritis synovium to illustrate the lining (*) and sublining layers. CD68 staining demonstrates type A (macrophage-like) synoviocytes (brown stain), which are prominent in the lining layer. The other cells in the lining layer (blue) are type B (fibroblastic) synoviocytes. There is again prominent neovascularization in the sublining. Original magnification x 20. Image courtesy of Dr J. Canete.

the articular cartilage, where the secretion of cytokines and cartilage- and bone-degrading enzymes results in the characteristic destructive changes of RA. The invading synovium is termed pannus, and the zone of invasion is called the cartilage–pannus junction. Similar changes to these occur in the synovium lining tendons and bursae, and several of the deformities characteristic of RA result from the weakening and rupture of tendons by inflamed synovium.

Inflammatory mediators

Pro-inflammatory cytokines are abundant in the RA synovium. Prominent among these are tumor necrosis factor (TNF), interleukin (IL)-1 and IL-6, but many others are present, including IL-12, IL-15, IL-17 and IL-18. The RA joint also contains anti-inflammatory cytokines, such as IL-10, IL-13 and transforming growth factor β (TGFβ), as well as high levels of cytokine-neutralizing factors, such as soluble TNF receptors and IL-1 receptor antagonist (IL-1ra). These data suggest that a cytokine imbalance, in favor of pro-inflammatory mediators, may be a key pathogenic mechanism in RA (Figure 3.4). A search for pivotal regulatory cytokines suggested that synovial TNF could orchestrate the expression of other pro-inflammatory mediators, and subsequent studies in animal models and then in humans have shown TNF blockade to be a useful therapeutic strategy for RA (see

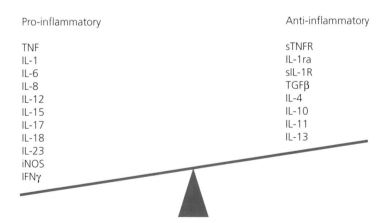

Pro-inflammatory	Anti-inflammatory
TNF	sTNFR
IL-1	IL-1ra
IL-6	sIL-1R
IL-8	TGFβ
IL-12	IL-4
IL-15	IL-10
IL-17	IL-11
IL-18	IL-13
IL-23	
iNOS	
IFNγ	

Figure 3.4 The cytokine imbalance in rheumatoid arthritis. IFNγ, interferon γ; IL, interleukin; IL-1ra, interleukin-1 receptor antagonist; iNOS, inducible nitric oxide synthase; sIL-1R, soluble IL-1 receptor; sTNFR, soluble TNF receptor; TGFβ, tissue growth factor β; TNF, tumor necrosis factor.

Chapter 9). Recently, however, IL-6 receptor blockade has proved to be as effective, emphasizing the complex interplay between distinct inflammatory mediators in RA. Other pro-inflammatory factors present within the RA synovium include the pleiotropic mediator nitric oxide, prostaglandins, leukotrienes and reactive oxygen intermediates. The accumulation of the last of these has been attributed to a form of reperfusion injury within the chronically inflamed joint secondary to elevated intra-articular pressure. The consequent hypoxia is one of a number of stimuli reported to promote neovascularization in rheumatoid synovitis. Others include soluble factors such as vascular endothelial growth factor (VEGF) and soluble vascular cell adhesion molecule-1 (VCAM-1), which stimulate endothelial cell growth.

Cellular infiltrates

Despite their central role in RA symptomatology, pro-inflammatory cytokine production is unlikely to be the primary abnormality in RA. For example, cell-to-cell contact between activated T cells and synovial monocytes is a stimulus to TNF production and the rheumatoid synovium is heavily infiltrated with a variety of immune and inflammatory cells.

Recently, the importance of different T cell subsets in RA has been revisited. T helper (TH)17 cells, physiologically important in the fight against extracellular bacterial infections, appear pivotal in the pathogenesis of inflammatory diseases such as RA. The 'signature' cytokine of this subset, IL-17, has pleiotropic actions relevant to RA: endothelial cell activation, induction of pro-inflammatory cytokine secretion (TNF, IL-1, IL-6 and IL-8), and RANKL induction on chondrocytes and osteoblasts, leading to osteoclast activation. These actions contribute to synovial inflammation as well as bone damage and resorption. Another important T cell subset is the FoxP3-transcription-factor-positive regulatory subset. Individuals congenitally lacking these cells suffer catastrophic autoimmunity and a number of studies have demonstrated qualitative and/or quantitative abnormalities in RA. The relative balance between TH17 and T regulatory cell (Treg) activity can be influenced by the local cytokine environment and there is some evidence for interconversion between the two subsets under certain conditions. There is less evidence for prominent involvement of the more traditional TH1 and TH2 cell subsets in RA pathogenesis.

The role of B cells in rheumatoid synovitis has been revisited in recent years. In addition to producing autoantibodies, B cells secrete pro-inflammatory cytokines (including TNF and IL-6), and are also efficient antigen-presenting cells. There is good evidence that autoantibodies such as anti-citrullinated peptide antibody (ACPA; see page 61) are produced locally in rheumatoid synovium, within the lymphoid follicles, and B cell depletion is now an established and effective therapy for RA (see Chapter 9). Macrophages are almost certainly the major 'factory' for pro-inflammatory cytokines in RA, and recently there has been renewed interest in the potential role of mast cells in the disease. Dendritic cells are the 'generals' of the immune system that, in large part, determine the outcome of T cell differentiation. They are also present in rheumatoid synovium and could play an important role in disease pathogenesis.

Homing of cells to synovium

A number of adhesion molecules are abundant on the vascular endothelium in rheumatoid synovium, including E-selectin and intercellular adhesion molecules (ICAMs). Their expression is stimulated by pro-inflammatory cytokines, such as IL-1, TNF and IL-17, and results in the recruitment of inflammatory cells via counter-receptors such as the integrin leukocyte function-associated molecule-1 (LFA-1) and very late activation antigen-4 (VLA-4). Further progress of inflammatory cells into the joint is stimulated by chemokines, of which there is an abundance in the rheumatoid synovium. These include monocyte chemotactic protein-1 (MCP-1 [also known as chemokine {C-C motif} ligand 2 or CCL2]), IL-8 (also known as C-X-C motif chemokine ligand 8 or CXCL8), regulated upon activation, normally T expressed, and presumably secreted (RANTES [also known as chemokine {C-C motif} ligand 5 or CCL5]), monocyte chemoattractant protein 4 (MCP-4 [chemokine {C-C motif} ligand 13 or CCL13]), stromal cell-derived factor 1 (SDF-1 [also known as

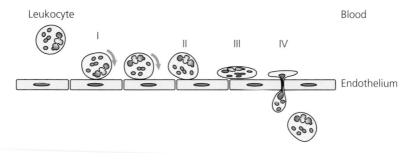

Figure 3.5 The stages of leukocyte migration into an inflammatory site. (I) Rolling along activated endothelium, mediated by selectin–selectin-ligand interactions. (II) Slowing and activation of leukocytes, mediated by endothelially located chemokines and by integrin–ligand interactions. (III) Tethering and flattening of leukocytes, mediated by integrin–ligand interactions. (IV) Transmigration of leukocytes, along a chemokine gradient and guided by integrin–connective-tissue–ligand interactions.

chemokine {C-X-C motif} ligand 12 or CXCL12]), macrophage inflammatory protein 1 α (MIP-1-α [also known as chemokine {C-C motif} ligand 3 or CCL3) and fractalkine (chemokine [C-X3-C motif] ligand 1 or CX3CL1). These low-molecular-weight peptides provide activating and chemotactic stimuli for inflammatory cells (Figure 3.5).

Immunosenescence

The RA immune system has several similarities to the aged human immune system (immunosenescence): thymic function is impaired and lymphocyte telomeres are shortened. Several lymphocyte subsets – some of which appear to be constitutively activated – resemble those found in elderly individuals. Whether these changes are the consequence of chronic inflammation or an integral aspect of disease pathogenesis remains to be proven, although several of these abnormalities can be found in early disease.

Apoptosis

Physiological tissue hyperplasia and lymphocyte proliferation during immune responses are normally counteracted by programmed cell death, or apoptosis, preventing an overaccumulation of cells.

Relatively few apoptotic cells are present in rheumatoid synovium, however, despite pro-apoptotic stimuli such as hypoxia and TNF. That apoptosis is actively inhibited is substantiated by the abundance of anti-apoptotic molecules, such as sentrin in synovial lining cells and BCL2-like 1 (BCL2L1, also known as Bcl-xL) in synovial lymphocytes. Soluble anti-apoptotic molecules such as soluble Fas ligand (sCD95L) and osteoprotegerin are also present within the RA joint. In a complex interplay, type B synoviocytes also secrete growth factors that inhibit apoptosis of lymphocytes, such as BAFF (also known as TNF [ligand] superfamily member 13b or TNFSF13B) which maintains B cell survival and interferon (IFN)-β which prevents T cell apoptosis. Impaired synoviocyte apoptosis may also result from mutation of protective oncogenes, such as p53, possibly secondary to the hypoxic intra-articular environment, and is central to the synoviocyte model of RA pathogenesis (see page 34).

Cartilage and bone destruction

A variety of destructive enzymes are secreted by rheumatoid pannus. Prominent among these are the various matrix metalloproteinases (MMPs) – which include collagenases, stromelysins and gelatinases – and serine and cysteine proteases, such as cathepsins. These enzymes act upon collagen and the proteoglycan matrix, thereby destroying the central structure of articular cartilage. As with the cytokines, these enzymes are controlled by physiological inhibitors such as tissue inhibitors of metalloproteinases (TIMPs), again raising the possibility of a critical imbalance in RA synovium.

Osteoimmunology is a relatively new field that studies the interactions between the immune system and bone. Bone destruction in RA is mediated by osteoclasts, which differentiate from monocyte precursors. A critically important molecule in this regard is receptor activator of nuclear factor κB ligand [RANKL] (Figure 3.6). This is a transmembrane protein induced on fibroblast-like synoviocytes (FLS) and osteoblasts by pro-inflammatory cytokines, and a soluble form is secreted by activated T cells. By interacting with membrane receptor activator of nuclear factor κB (RANK) on osteoclast precursors, RANKL results in their differentiation and activation, ultimately

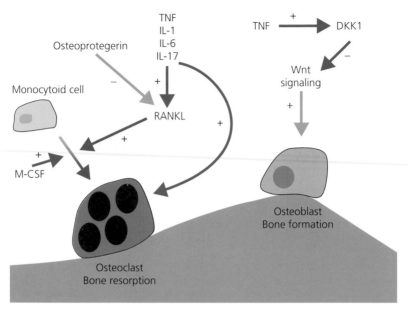

Figure 3.6 Bone formation and resorption in rheumatoid arthritis (RA). Bone destruction is mediated by osteoclasts, which differentiate from monocytoid cells under the influence of receptor activator of nuclear factor κB ligand (RANKL) and macrophage colony-stimulating factor (M-CSF). RANKL exists in a soluble form, secreted by activated T cells, and a transmembrane form induced on fibroblast-like synoviocytes and osteoblasts. Osteoprotegerin, a natural antagonist, appears insufficient to neutralize RANKL in RA. Interleukin (IL)-1, IL-6, IL-17 and tumor necrosis factor (TNF) induce RANKL expression and also activate osteoclasts directly. Bone formation is mediated by osteoblasts under the influence of Wnt signaling. In RA, TNF stimulates Dickkopf-1 (DKK1), which inhibits the Wnt pathway. Consequently in RA the net balance is unopposed bone resorption. Wnt, wingless-related MMTV integration site mouse mammary tumor virus [MMTV] family. Pink arrows illustrate bone resorptive stimuli, blue arrows counter-resorptive or bone formative stimuli.

leading to bone destruction. Macrophage colony stimulating factor (M-CSF) is also necessary for osteoclast formation, whereas TNF, IL-1, IL-6 and IL-17 induce RANKL production, all contributing to both the periarticular and systemic osteoporosis characteristic of RA.

Osteoprotegerin (also known as tumor necrosis factor receptor superfamily member 11B [TNFRSF11B]) is a decoy receptor that physiologically protects osteoclasts from the actions of RANKL, but which appears to be overwhelmed in RA. The lack of counterbalancing bone formation in RA has recently been attributed to downregulation of Wnt signaling, which is important for osteoblast formation (Wnt derives from 'wingless-related MMTV integration site mouse mammary tumor virus [MMTV]' family). This is secondary to TNF-induced Dickkopf-1 (DKK1) production, which suppresses Wnt signaling.

A further relevant aspect of osteoimmunology relates to the recognition that the synovium can communicate with bone marrow via cortical bone channels. This may partly underlie bone edema present in early RA, which also contributes to periarticular bone loss. Furthermore, bone marrow provides niches for autoantibody-secreting B cells and plasma cells in RA.

Extra-articular disease

Less is understood about the pathogenesis of extra-articular RA, such as rheumatoid nodules, and inflammation of the pericardium, pleura and lung parenchyma (Chapter 5). None of these sites contains synovial tissue. Histology of rheumatoid nodules reveals pallisading macrophages surrounding a necrotic core, and scattered peripheral lymphocytes. Rheumatoid factor (RF; see page 60) and, in particular, small immune complexes composed of immunoglobulin (Ig)G RF dimers have been invoked to explain the extra-articular manifestations of RA. This hypothesis suggests that IgG RFs self-associate head to tail (Figure 3.7) and diffuse into the circulation and subsequently into the tissues. There they activate macrophages expressing Fcγ receptors (receptors for IgG), which then produce pro-inflammatory cytokines and chemokines, leading to further inflammatory cell influx. In contrast to RF, ACPAs have not been directly linked to RA pathogenesis, although they can contribute to synovitis in animal models of RA.

Rheumatoid vasculitis usually occurs in association with high levels of circulating IgM RF, which is highly effective at activating

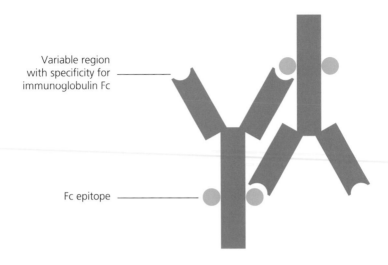

Variable region
with specificity for
immunoglobulin Fc

Fc epitope

Figure 3.7 The self-association of rheumatoid factors. Sites of extra-articular rheumatoid arthritis contain macrophages expressing CD16 (FcgγRIIIa). It has been hypothesized that rheumatoid factor dimers bind CD16 at these sites and activate the macrophages, resulting in inflammation.

complement. Deposition of IgM RF-containing immune complexes within the perivascular tissues may therefore lead to inflammation and hence vasculitis. The presence of cryoglobulins (RFs that precipitate at low temperatures) may lead to severe Raynaud's phenomenon and even necrosis and gangrene of the digits.

Cardiovascular disease
Cardiovascular disease (CVD) has been a well-recognized complication of RA for decades and accounts for at least 50% of the excess mortality seen in RA patients. Traditional risk factors (smoking, diabetes, hypertension, obesity and hyperlipidemia) cannot account for all of the excess CVD in RA and it is likely that inflammation and thrombogenic factors also contribute. Furthermore, it is now recognized that the pathology of atherosclerosis bears many resemblances to that of RA, in terms of cellular and pro-inflammatory mediators, as well as in the destructive enzymes that result in plaque

rupture. Therefore, whether enhanced atherosclerosis is purely secondary to RA manifestations or intrinsically linked to its pathogenesis awaits further study. However, cardiovascular complications can occur in early RA, before downstream sequelae such as joint damage. Ultimately, RA may (and should) become generally recognized as a predisposing factor for atherosclerosis in much the same way as diabetes mellitus is currently.

Neurological involvement and the hypothalamo–pituitary–adrenal axis

The symmetry of RA is highly suggestive of a neurological component to the disease, and RA synovium contains high levels of particular neuropeptides such as substance P. Furthermore, there is reduction in sympathetic innervations to the rheumatoid joint and local disruption of sex hormone metabolism and receptor expression. The relationship of these changes to the disease process remains unclear, but is reinforced by observations that include the sparing of paralyzed limbs in patients with neurological disorders such as strokes.

There is also evidence to support abnormalities in both the hypothalamo–pituitary–adrenal (HPA) and hypothalamo–pituitary–gonadal (HPG) axes in RA, including a suppressed response to stressful stimuli. Intrinsic HPA defects can also be demonstrated in some RA patients in response to conventional pharmacological stimuli.

Models of pathogenesis

A number of competing models attempt to consolidate the foregoing features.

The autoimmune model, now strongly supported by the results of genome-wide association studies (GWAS), views RA as a classic T-cell-mediated autoimmune disease, precipitated by autoreactivity against a joint component. Putative autoantigens include: type II collagen and aggrecan, components of articular cartilage; gp39, a protein produced by chondrocytes and synoviocytes; and a B-cell-derived protein called BiP (Ig heavy-chain-binding protein), which is an endoplasmic reticulum chaperonin. Post-translationally modified peptides, particularly citrullinated derivatives of joint autoantigen such as fibrinogen, collagen, vimentin and alpha-enolase, are also under intense scrutiny. With their evolutionarily conserved structure from microbes to man, heat shock proteins are also candidate autoantigens. The efficacy of immunosuppressive drugs such as ciclosporin (previously cyclosporin[e] A) and leflunomide and, in particular, the recent success of targeted therapeutic approaches such as costimulation blockade and B-cell depletion (see Chapter 9), attest to the importance of lymphocytes in disease pathogenesis.

A competing theory states that RA is primarily a disease of FLS. These cells are present in pannus and secrete many destructive factors. Furthermore, RA synovial fibroblasts exhibit characteristics reminiscent of malignant cells, such as upregulation of oncogenes, and the ability for prolonged growth with reduced contact inhibition in vitro. Recent experiments even suggest a propensity of these cells to migrate via the blood stream, potentially explaining the spread of RA to new joint areas. Thus, an intrinsic defect of these cells could explain many of the pathological features of RA, with chronic inflammation as a secondary phenomenon. The intercellular adhesion molecule cadherin-11 has been shown to be important for synovial membrane formation and to contribute to the abnormal behavior of RA FLS. On the other hand, it is equally plausible that abnormal FLS behavior is triggered by chronic autoimmunity and inflammation. Indeed, early and effective treatment of RA results in a less aggressive phenotype in terms of joint damage and destruction, suggesting that early suppression of inflammation may modulate the propensity of fibroblasts to destroy joints and soft tissue. The substrate for such an effect is unclear, but the new science of epigenetics could hold the key. Epigenetics refers to (heritable) changes in cell phenotype or gene expression that are unrelated to changes in the underlying DNA sequence. Many of the characteristics of the RA FLS could be explained by epigenetic influences of chronic inflammation.

Lastly, macrophages are abundant in synovium during the earliest stages of RA. They secrete TNF, IL-1 and IL-6, three of the pivotal cytokines in RA, and studies have shown a correlation between the number of synovial macrophages and the degree of joint destruction. Macrophages are also a good biomarker of therapeutic response to a variety of drugs. Thus, an intrinsic defect of these cells could underlie RA pathogenesis, although they are most readily implicated as essential players in the other models.

With the data emerging from GWAS, the autoimmune model appears most robust. Furthermore, the appearance of autoantibodies many years before disease onset (see page 18) also emphasizes immune dysregulation as the primary event in RA. Fibroblast and macrophage abnormalities may then follow as downstream sequelae.

Key points – pathogenesis

- Rheumatoid arthritis (RA) is a disease initially localized to the joint lining.
- Dominant features are synovial inflammation, and proliferation and outgrowth of the synovial lining layer, with destruction of articular cartilage and bone.
- Pro-inflammatory cytokines play a pivotal role in RA pathology.
- The primary pathogenic event may reside within the immune system or in the synovial lining. However, data from genome-wide association studies and preclinical autoantibody development suggest primary immune dysregulation.
- Accelerated cardiovascular disease in RA may be secondary to inflammation or intrinsic to the disease process.
- The inter-relationship between the immune system and bone is receiving increasing attention (osteoimmunology).

Key references

Bartok B, Firestein GS. Fibroblast-like synoviocytes: key effector cells in rheumatoid arthritis. *Immunol Rev* 2010;233:233–55.

Capellino S, Straub RH. Neuroendocrine immune pathways in chronic arthritis. *Best Pract Res Clin Rheumatol* 2008;22:285–97.

Chang SK, Gu Z, Brenner MB. Fibroblast-like synoviocytes in inflammatory arthritis pathology: the emerging role of cadherin-11. *Immunol Rev* 2010;233:256–66.

Cope AP. T cells in rheumatoid arthritis. *Arthritis Res Ther* 2008;10(suppl 1):S1.

Korb A, Pavenstadt H, Pap T. Cell death in rheumatoid arthritis. *Apoptosis* 2009;14:447–54.

Marston B, Palanichamy A, Anolik JH. B cells in the pathogenesis and treatment of rheumatoid arthritis. *Curr Opin Rheumatol* 2010;22: 307–15.

McInnes IB, Schett G. Cytokines in the pathogenesis of rheumatoid arthritis. *Nat Rev Immunol* 2007; 7:429–42.

Takayanagi H. Osteoimmunology and the effects of the immune system on bone. *Nat Rev Rheumatol* 2009; 5:667–76.

Turesson C, Matteson EL. Vasculitis in rheumatoid arthritis. *Curr Opin Rheumatol* 2009;21:35–40.

Weyand CM, Fujii H, Shao L, Goronzy JJ. Rejuvenating the immune system in rheumatoid arthritis. *Nat Rev Rheumatol* 2009;5:583–8.

Rheumatoid arthritis (RA) is the most common form of inflammatory arthritis and is a heterogeneous disease. There is no pathognomonic clinical sign or laboratory test, with diagnosis resting on a pattern of clinical and serological features. Classification criteria for RA have recently been updated jointly by the American College of Rheumatology (ACR) and European League Against Rheumatism (EULAR). Compared with the previous 1987 criteria, more emphasis is now placed on autoantibodies (rheumatoid factor [RF] and anti-citrullinated peptide antibody [ACPA]) and acute phase reactants (erythrocyte sedimentation rate [ESR] and C-reactive protein [CRP]) (see Chapter 5).

Incidence and prevalence

By definition, RA can start at any age from 16 upwards, although an equivalent disease also occurs in children (polyarticular juvenile idiopathic arthritis). The overall prevalence of RA in adults is 0.5–1% in most Western populations. It is two to three times more common in women than in men and its incidence increases with age. The incidence of RA varies by as much as tenfold between studies, and lies between 30 and 300 per 100 000 population per year. There is a suggestion that the incidence is declining, particularly in women, which some have linked to a protective effect of the oral contraceptive pill, though this remains unproven.

The peak age of onset varies between studies but is probably in the fifth decade of life. RA occurs in all societies, with no clear geographic or climatic influence. On the other hand there is variation between communities. For example, there is a high prevalence (approximately 5%) in some Native American populations such as the Pima Indians. Similarly, a low prevalence has been reported in certain rural Chinese and Japanese communities. In Africa, a lower prevalence was reported in a rural than in an urban community. This could reflect a genuine difference in prevalence but could also be explained by other factors, such as a lower mortality from RA-associated infections in the town-dwellers or differences in the age structure of the two communities.

Mortality

Historically, RA has been considered a chronic disabling disease that does not shorten lifespan. This is untrue, however, and various studies have reported a standardized mortality ratio of between 1.3 and 3.0 compared with the general population. Consequently, life expectancy in severe RA is reduced, on average, by 7 years for men and 4 years for women. Furthermore, the improvement in life expectancy seen in the general population over recent years does not appear to have extended to the RA population, resulting in a widening gap in mortality rates (Figure 4.1).

The causes of death are largely those prevalent in society as a whole, such as ischemic heart disease, infections and malignancies. RA patients are more than three times more likely to be hospitalized with a myocardial infarction (MI) than patients without RA and almost six times more likely to have a silent MI. RA patients are also twice as likely to develop heart failure, even allowing for traditional risk factors and ischemic heart disease. Clinical and subclinical inflammation probably provide the critical risk factors for ischemic heart disease although this remains to be definitively proven, particularly because atherosclerosis itself has an inflammatory pathogenesis (see Chapter 3). Subclinical vasculitis could also predispose to atherosclerosis in RA. It is noteworthy that comorbidities often present atypically in RA, and are associated with greater mortality; for example, MI is more likely to present silently, and heart failure with preserved ejection fraction.

The overall malignancy risk in RA is similar to that in the general population, although there is a slight increase in immune system neoplasms such as lymphomas (approximately twice as common in RA) and multiple myeloma. Lung cancer is also increased in RA, presumably because smoking is a risk factor for the disease, whereas colorectal cancer is reduced, probably reflecting a protective effect of non-steroidal anti-inflammatory drugs (NSAIDs).

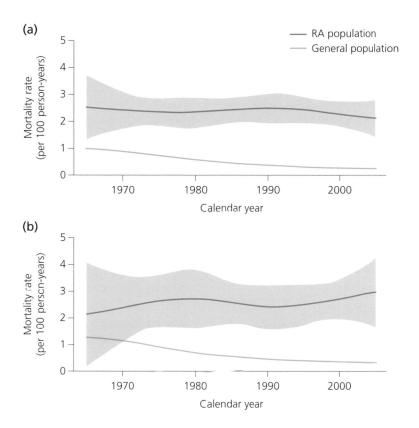

Figure 4.1 Mortality rates in rheumatoid arthritis compared with the general population: (a) women; and (b) men (populations from Minnesota, USA). Adapted with permission from Gonzalez et al., 2007.

Infection-related mortality is increased in RA. In part this is secondary to immunosuppressive drug therapy (particularly corticosteroids) and chronic ill health but there is also evidence for suppressed immunity even in early disease, potentially linked to the effects of chronically elevated levels of tumor necrosis factor (TNF).

As well as predisposing to local infections and contributing to the enhanced lung cancer risk, interstitial lung disease per se is a cause of excess mortality in RA patients, as is peptic ulcer disease, the latter largely secondary to NSAID and corticosteroid use.

Some recent studies have suggested that early intervention with antirheumatic drugs such as methotrexate and TNF blockade has reduced the overall severity of RA, with a concomitant reduction in mortality. More studies are required to provide a definitive answer, however, particularly within the context of the lack of overall reduction in mortality seen in general epidemiological studies.

Economic impact

The economic costs of an illness are categorized as direct, indirect and intangible. Direct costs are the costs of medicines, and primary and secondary care. For RA, these include the costs of inpatient care, either for rehabilitation or for complications of the disease and joint surgery. Indirect costs represent the consequences of unemployment and reduced productivity. Intangible costs reflect the psychosocial consequences of RA that impact on psychological wellbeing and quality of life. A recent analysis by the UK National Audit Office estimated the annual direct costs of RA to be in the region of £560 million, and total costs up to £4.8 billion per year. The direct costs divide approximately equally between primary and secondary care, with an increasing proportion of spend attributable to biological therapies (£160 million annually).

Work disability in RA varies between studies, but functional disability invariably occurs in the absence of early and effective treatment. A UK-based study from the pre-biologic era, of patients with disease of an average duration of 6 months, reported only 33% of patients with normal function at presentation and 10% of patients with severe disability. By 5 years, 40% had normal function, but 16% had severe disability. Of those initially in paid employment, 27% were work-disabled by 5 years. Notably, 17% had already undergone orthopedic surgery by that time. Other studies suggest an even higher rate of work disability, with a third of patients ceasing work within 2 years of diagnosis, although early biological therapy has had a major impact on job retention and employment prospects.

The cost–benefit equation. Several of the newer therapies for RA have been expensive to develop and are costly to manufacture;

consequently, their price can exceed \$15 000 (£10 000)/patient/year. Furthermore, some require intravenous administration, which entails additional costs. If efficacy is high, however, the need for other therapies and surgery should be reduced. If, in addition, function and employment are retained, total direct, indirect and intangible costs will be significantly reduced. A recent estimate from the UK National Rheumatoid Arthritis Society suggests that the loss of productivity when a patient stops work because of RA equates to almost £300 000.

Thus, the cost–benefit equation for novel RA interventions is complicated and cannot be fully ascertained for several years after their introduction into clinical practice. A corollary is the importance of adequate documentation of outcomes in patients receiving such treatments, particularly indicators of function, quality of life and participation (see Chapter 7). Such data may be critical in the ultimate acceptance of innovative but expensive interventions of any type in cost-conscious and resource-finite healthcare systems.

Key points – epidemiology

- Rheumatoid arthritis (RA) is a global disease, present in all populations studied.
- RA should not be viewed as a benign chronic disease of the elderly. The peak age of onset occurs during working life, severely reducing participation and productivity. Furthermore, mortality is increased and there is very significant comorbidity.
- The disease inflicts huge economic costs on both the individual and society. It is essential that total healthcare and societal costs are considered when the economic impact of new drugs is considered.
- It remains to be determined whether the new targeted biological therapies will reduce the mortality associated with RA.

Key references

Gabriel SE, Michaud K. Epidemiological studies in incidence, prevalence, mortality, and comorbidity of the rheumatic diseases. *Arthritis Res Ther* 2009;11:229.

Gonzalez A, Maradit Kremers H, Crowson CS et al. The widening mortality gap between rheumatoid arthritis patients and the general population. *Arthritis Rheum* 2007;56:3583–7.

Michaud K, Wolfe F. Comorbidities in rheumatoid arthritis. *Best Pract Res Clin Rheumatol* 2007;21: 885–906.

National Audit Office. *Services for People with Rheumatoid Arthritis.* London: The Stationery Office, 2009. Available from www.nao.org.uk/publications/0809/services_for_people_with_rheum.aspx, last accessed 8 Nov 2010.

Naz SM, Symmons DP. Mortality in established rheumatoid arthritis. *Best Pract Res Clin Rheumatol* 2007;21:871–83.

Schoels M, Wong J, Scott DL et al. Economic aspects of treatment options in rheumatoid arthritis: a systematic literature review informing the EULAR recommendations for the management of rheumatoid arthritis. *Ann Rheum Dis* 2010;69:995–1003.

Sokka T, Abelson B, Pincus T. Mortality in rheumatoid arthritis: 2008 update. *Clin Exp Rheumatol* 2008;26:S35–61.

Sokka T, Kautiainen H, Pincus T et al. Work disability remains a major problem in rheumatoid arthritis in the 2000s: data from 32 countries in the QUEST-RA study. *Arthritis Res Ther* 2010; 12:R42.

Young A. What have we learnt from early rheumatoid arthritis cohorts? *Best Pract Res Clin Rheumatol* 2009;23:3–12

The pathological and etiologic heterogeneity of rheumatoid arthritis (RA) is reflected clinically, and RA can be difficult to diagnose in its earliest stages. Guidance from the UK's National Institute for Health and Clinical Excellence (NICE) states: "refer for specialist opinion any person with suspected persistent synovitis of undetermined cause. Refer urgently if any of the following apply: the small joints of the hands or feet are affected; more than one joint is affected; there has been a delay of 3 months or longer between onset of symptoms and seeking medical advice".

Early disease
There are no pathognomonic clinical or laboratory features of RA, and there are a number of potential differential diagnoses (Table 5.1).

The diagnosis of RA rests on the presence of a constellation of clinical and laboratory features. The 1987 American College of Rheumatology revised classification criteria (Table 5.2) have been superseded by the 2010 American College of Rheumatology (ACR)/ European League Against Rheumatism (EULAR) criteria (Table 5.3). The new criteria attempt to ascertain the likelihood of developing persistent damaging joint inflammation that requires therapy in patients with recent-onset synovitis. They are weighted and place more emphasis on the number of involved joints and pattern of joint involvement, the presence and titer of autoantibodies (rheumatoid factor [RF] and anti-citrullinated peptide antibody [ACPA]) and elevated inflammatory markers (erythrocyte sedimentation rate [ESR] or C-reactive protein [CRP]). Early morning joint stiffness, subcutaneous nodules and radiographic features have been dropped from the criteria. A tree algorithm can also be used to classify RA (Figure 5.1).

The most common joints to be affected by RA at presentation are the metacarpophalangeal (MCP) and proximal interphalangeal (PIP) joints of the hands, and the metatarsophalangeal (MTP) joints of the

TABLE 5.1

Differential diagnosis of recent-onset polyarthritis or polyarthralgia

Inflammatory synovitis
- Rheumatoid arthritis
- Psoriatic arthritis
- Enteropathic arthritis
- Reactive arthritis
- Reiter's syndrome
- Ankylosing spondylitis
- Post-viral arthritis
- Inflammatory osteoarthritis
- Polyarticular gout
- Pseudogout
- Connective tissue disease (e.g. systemic lupus erythematosus, systemic sclerosis)
- Vasculitis (e.g. Wegener's granulomatosis, Henoch–Schönlein purpura)
- Sarcoidosis
- Behçet's disease

Non-inflammatory conditions
- Generalized osteoarthritis
- Fibromyalgia

Metabolic and endocrine conditions
- Osteomalacia
- Hyperparathyroidism
- Renal bone disease (in chronic renal impairment)
- Hypothyroidism

Chronic infections
- Subacute bacterial endocarditis
- Hepatitis B
- Human immunodeficiency virus
- Lyme disease (in endemic areas)

Miscellaneous conditions
- Paraneoplastic syndromes
- Multiple myeloma
- Polymyalgia rheumatica
- Septic arthritis (not usually polyarticular)

feet. In addition to pain and swelling, early morning stiffness of affected joint areas is highly characteristic. Reflecting the overnight accumulation of inflammatory fluid within the joints, stiffness usually lasts for at least 30 minutes but may not resolve for several hours. This distribution of joint involvement results in early functional

TABLE 5.2

1987 American College of Rheumatology classification criteria for rheumatoid arthritis

A patient must have at least four of the following:

- Morning stiffness in and around joints lasting ≥ 1 hour before maximal improvement, for at least 6 weeks
- Soft tissue swelling (arthritis) of ≥ 3 joint areas, for at least 6 weeks
- Swelling (arthritis) of the proximal interphalangeal, metacarpophalangeal or wrist joints, for at least 6 weeks
- Symmetrical arthritis, for at least 6 weeks
- Subcutaneous nodules
- Positive test for rheumatoid factor
- Radiographic erosions and/or periarticular osteopenia in hand and/or wrist joints

impairment and slowed mobility, to which excessive fatigue and malaise may contribute. Objectively, there may be swelling of affected joints, which can be accentuated by inflammation of overlying tendon sheaths, particularly in the hands. Range of joint motion is restricted by synovitis of both the joints themselves and the tendon sheaths.

While this is the most common presentation of RA, there are many other possibilities. The disease can affect any synovial joint, and larger joints such as the elbows, shoulders or knees may also be involved. Unusual symptoms reflect the involvement of joints such as the crico-arytenoid joint of the larynx, with resultant hoarseness. Inflammation of synovium at extra-articular sites leads to tenosynovitis and bursitis. Tenosynovitis further compounds functional impairment, particularly of the hands and wrists. Bursitis causes pain at juxta-articular sites: for example, at the hip, where trochanteric bursitis is common. The tempo of onset is also variable, ranging from an acute dramatic presentation in up to one-third of cases to the classic insidious clinical picture, where symptoms may have been present for weeks or months before the patient sought

TABLE 5.3

2010 ACR/EULAR classification criteria for rheumatoid arthritis

Clinical finding	Score
*Joint involvement**	(0–5)
1 large joint[†]	0
2–10 large joints[†]	1
1–3 small joints[‡] (± large joint involvement)	2
4–10 small joints[‡] (± large joint involvement)	3
> 10 joints[§] (with at least one small joint)	5
*Serology[¶]***	(0–3)
Negative RF and negative ACPA	0
Low positive RF or low positive ACPA	2
High positive RF or high positive ACPA	3
*Acute phase reactants***[††]	(0–1)
Normal CRP and normal ESR	0
Abnormal CRP or abnormal ESR	1
Duration of symptoms[‡‡]	(0–1)
< 6 weeks	0
≥ 6 weeks	1

For the criteria to be applied there must be at least one joint with definite clinical synovitis (swelling), which is not better explained by another disease. To be classified with RA a patient must score at least 6 points. A patient with synovitis and a lower score, without a clear alternative diagnosis (see Table 5.1), is classified as having an undifferentiated arthritis.
*Joint involvement refers to any swollen or tender joint on examination, which may be confirmed by imaging evidence of synovitis. Distal interphalangeal joints, 1st carpometacarpal joint and 1st metatarsophalangeal joint are excluded from assessment. Categories of joint distribution are classified according to the location and number of involved joints, with placement into the highest category possible based on the pattern of joint involvement.
†Medium to large joints are the shoulders, elbows, hips, knees and ankles.
‡Small joints are the metacarpophalangeal joints, proximal interphalangeal joints, metatarsophalangeal joints 2–5, thumb interphalangeal joints and wrists.

CONTINUED

TABLE 5.3 (CONTINUED)

§At least one of the involved joints must be a small joint; the other joints can include any combination of large and additional small joints, as well as other joints not specifically listed elsewhere (e.g. temporomandibular, acromioclavicular, sternoclavicular).

¶Negative refers to IU values ≤ ULN for the laboratory and assay; low positive refers to IU values that are > ULN but ≤ 3× ULN for the laboratory and assay; high positive refers to IU values that are > 3× the ULN for the laboratory and assay. Where RF information is only available as positive or negative, a positive result should be scored as low positive for RF.

**Individuals should only be scored by these criteria if at least one test result is available. Where a value for a serological test or acute-phase reactant is not available, that test should be considered as negative/normal.

††Normal/abnormal is determined by local laboratory standards.

‡‡Duration of symptoms refers to patient self-report of the duration of signs or symptoms of synovitis (e.g. pain, swelling, tenderness) of joints that are clinically involved at the time of assessment, regardless of treatment status.

ACPA, anti-citrullinated peptide antibody; ACR, American College of Rheumatology; CRP, C-reactive protein; ESR, erythrocyte sedimentation rate; EULAR, European League Against Rheumatism; IU, international unit; RF, rheumatoid factor; ULN, upper limit of normal.

medical advice. Fatigue and malaise may be prominent features and, in some cases, may overshadow the articular symptoms.

The course of early disease is also variable, ranging from progressive unremitting symptoms spreading to additional joints to less common 'palindromic' symptoms, which may last from just hours to days before remitting, only to reappear at a later date. In the elderly, prominent myalgia may add to diagnostic confusion and some individuals present with symptoms indistinguishable from polymyalgia rheumatica before evolving to more typical RA. In such patients, the coexistence of myalgic and arthritic symptoms further compounds disability.

Established rheumatoid arthritis

The picture of established RA is changing as a result of effective therapies being used earlier in the disease. Thus, the signs may be similar to those of early disease, although more joints generally become affected as the disease becomes established. The classic hallmarks of established RA are less commonly seen today, but are the characteristic deformities that result from a combination of synovitis and resultant joint damage, tenosynovitis and ligamentous laxity (Figure 5.2 [see also Figure 5.6]).

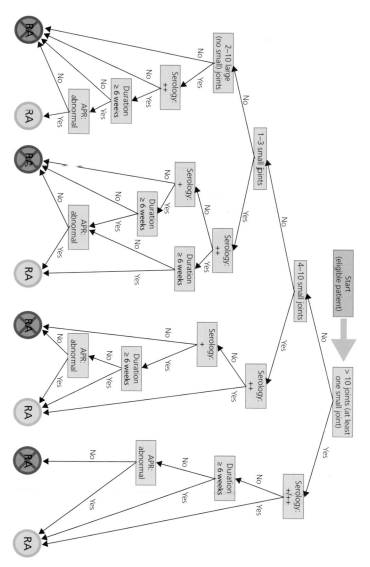

Figure 5.1 Tree algorithm for classifying definite rheumatoid arthritis (RA) (green circles) or for excluding its current presence (red circles) among those who are eligible to be assessed by the new criteria. APR, acute-phase response; serology +, low positive for rheumatoid factor (RF) or anti-citrullinated peptide antibodies (ACPAs); serology ++, high positive for RF or ACPA; serology +/++, serology either + or ++. See footnotes to Table 5.3 for further explanation of categories.

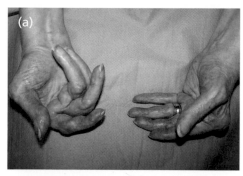

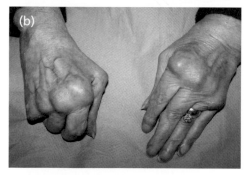

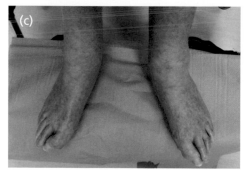

Figure 5.2 Characteristic appearance of the hands and feet in rheumatoid arthritis. (a, b) The hands demonstrate: swelling, subluxation and ulnar deviation at the metacarpophalangeal joints; flexion deformities of the fingers and Z deformity of the thumb on the right; and early swan neck deformities on the left. Multiple rheumatoid nodules are also evident, as is (teno)synovitis at the right wrist. (c) The feet demonstrate swelling and valgus deformities at the ankles, flattening of the longitudinal arches with pes planus, and early clawing of the toes.

Hands. In the hands, the swan-neck, boutonnière and z thumb deformities represent tendon slippage with an altered axis of traction that compromises joint motion. Subluxation and ulnar deviation at the MCP joints, and subluxation at the wrist are also characteristic features of established RA. Flexor tenosynovitis is additionally associated with 'triggering' (locking or 'catching') of the fingers.

Feet. In the feet, the subtalar joint and talonavicular joint are more commonly affected than the ankle joint itself. A valgus deformity at the subtalar joint and associated ligamentous laxity results in flattening of the longitudinal arch and pes planus. Disease of the MTP joints and associated tendons results in splaying and clawing of the toes, followed by subluxation. Consequent pressure on the metatarsal heads during walking results in the characteristic symptom of 'walking on pebbles'. When examining the feet, inspection of the plantar surface may reveal calluses, under the metatarsal heads and at other sites, suggesting impaired foot mechanics.

Neuromuscular complications. In established RA, there is significant muscle wasting around affected joints. In the upper limbs, this may be prominent in the hands and forearms, compounded by cervical spine disease and associated radiculopathy or by compression neuropathies.

RA can affect the cervical spine at any level, leading to various sequelae. The best known, although not the most common, is atlanto-axial subluxation. This arises from synovitis affecting the articulation between the odontoid peg of the axis and the transverse ligament of the atlas. The design of this articulation enables rotatory movement but, with disruption of the transverse ligament, anterior–posterior movement also becomes possible with the danger of spinal cord compression by the odontoid peg during neck flexion (Figure 5.3). The peg may also separate from the axis completely and migrate cranially towards the foramen magnum, causing basilar invagination and compression of the cervical cord and medulla.

More commonly, synovitis of the apophyseal joints at lower cervical levels leads to subluxation and spinal cord compression. The resultant myelopathy is characterized by upper-limb symptoms and signs in a radicular distribution, alongside 'long tract' pyramidal and sensory features affecting the lower limbs. In some cases, cervical spine disease is relatively asymptomatic until the sudden appearance of neurological deficits. A high index of suspicion is therefore necessary, and surveillance radiology should be considered in patients with evidence of cervical spine RA, with a view to stabilization surgery for progressive subluxation at any level. The cervical spine is also

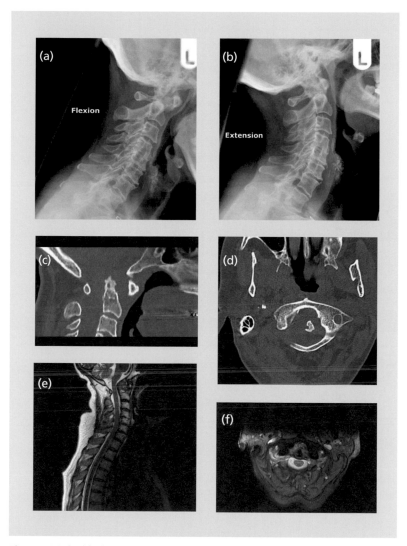

Figure 5.3 (a, b) Plain cervical spine radiographs of a patient with rheumatoid arthritis, demonstrating anterior subluxation of the atlas (C1) on flexion, with increased distance between the odontoid peg and anterior arch of the atlas. (c, d) The eroded and posteriorly migrated dens is clearly visible on sagittal and transverse CT scans. (e, f) Sagittal and transverse MRI scans demonstrate indentation of the spinal canal by inflammatory tissue at C1, as well as additional damage at the lower cervical levels. Images courtesy of Dr G. Hide.

vulnerable in RA patients undergoing laryngeal intubation as part of a general anesthetic, or requiring upper gastrointestinal endoscopy, and a full assessment is mandatory in such cases.

Entrapment neuropathies are also common causes of pain, neurological symptoms and muscle wasting in RA. By far the commonest is carpal tunnel syndrome due to median nerve compression by synovitis at the wrist, which may even be a presenting feature. Similarly, synovitis at the elbow can cause entrapment of the ulnar nerve or the posterior interosseous branch of the radial nerve, the latter causing wrist drop. Again, these features can severely compromise already-reduced hand function. At the ankle, entrapment of the medial peroneal nerve in the tarsal tunnel may cause pain or numbness of the medial border of the foot (tarsal tunnel syndrome).

In patients with rheumatoid vasculitis, involvement of the vasa nervorum may present as a 'glove-and-stocking' sensorimotor neuropathy.

Extra-articular features

Most extra-articular features of RA occur in RF-positive individuals with severe active joint disease. Occasionally, however, serious extra-articular involvement or even vasculitis arises in patients whose arthritis appears to have remitted or 'burnt out'. In particular, corneal 'melts' (see pages 55–6) frequently arise in elderly patients with minimal inflammatory joint symptoms. There is no obvious explanation for this paradox, which emphasizes the importance of regular and systematic review of RA patients by a specialist throughout the course of their disease.

Systemic features. The most common extra-articular manifestation is the rheumatoid nodule. These are usually subcutaneous and occur most commonly overlying pressure points. They are firm and non-tender unless infected, and range in size from a few millimeters in diameter to several centimeters. Common sites for nodules are the extensor surface of the forearms and over pressure points of the wrists, hands (see Figure 5.2a,b) and feet. Nodules may also occur at non-cutaneous sites. In the lungs, a solitary nodule may mimic a malignant tumor. In contrast, whilst less common now, massive and multiple nodules may be seen in ex-coal miners with pneumoconiosis (Caplan's syndrome). When localized to the sclera of the eye, nodules may cause thinning and, rarely, perforation of the globe (scleromalacia perforans). Nodules often improve with effective treatment of RA, but methotrexate may worsen nodulosis in some patients despite improvement in articular disease activity.

Lymphadenopathy is also associated with active RA and may coexist with systemic features such as fever and weight loss, raising the possibility of lymphoma. Histology, however, generally reveals 'reactive changes' of mild follicular hyperplasia.

Abnormal liver function tests are also a frequent finding in active RA, with mild and non-specific changes on liver biopsy. It is important to distinguish disease-related changes in these test results from abnormalities induced by therapies. This requires clinical judgment as well as careful monitoring of liver function tests in patients receiving potentially hepatotoxic therapies, such as methotrexate (see Chapter 8).

Amyloidosis, secondary to the deposition of serum amyloid A protein (an acute-phase reactant) in the tissues, is now a rare complication of RA, and reflects prolonged, active disease. It can present with multi-organ symptoms and signs, involving the kidney, intestines, liver, spleen and heart. Carpal tunnel syndrome is a more benign presentation.

Hematological complications. Active RA is often associated with anemia. This is usually normochromic and normocytic and a consequence of chronic inflammation. Hepcidin is released by the liver under the influence of interleukin (IL)-6, and inhibits iron release from macrophages as well as intestinal iron absorption. Iron deficiency may coexist, however, secondary to drug-induced gastrointestinal blood loss.

Other causes of anemia in RA include an autoimmune hemolytic anemia, which is uncommon, and drug-induced marrow suppression. In common with other inflammatory conditions, thrombocytosis may occur in active RA, secondary to IL-6-mediated megakaryocyte stimulation. In Felty's syndrome, patients with RA develop splenomegaly with features of hypersplenism (pancytopenia in the peripheral blood). Neutropenia is usually more marked than either thrombocytopenia or anemia. This is a serious complication, associated with recurrent bacterial infections, chronic leg ulcers and increased mortality. The etiology of Felty's syndrome is not understood, but some patients have an excess of natural killer (NK)-cell-like large granular lymphocytes in their peripheral blood.

Chest disease. Lung involvement is common in RA, with pleural disease being present in up to 50% of postmortem examinations. Patients may experience pleuritic chest pain and pleural effusions, but lung involvement is often asymptomatic. An inflammatory alveolitis (interstitial pneumonitis) is less common but can lead to irreversible pulmonary fibrosis if untreated. It generally starts in the lower lobes and presents as a dry cough, or as dyspnea on exertion. Other pulmonary manifestations include intrapulmonary nodules and obliterative bronchiolitis. The most serious of these in terms of mortality is diffuse pulmonary fibrosis.

In a community-based study, 6% of RA patients developed symptomatic interstitial lung disease within 10 years of disease onset. However, one study reported that 19% of unselected RA patients had alveolitis on high-resolution CT scan. RA-associated pulmonary fibrosis can be difficult to distinguish from pulmonary toxicity secondary to drugs such as methotrexate and leflunomide.

Serositis is also a common postmortem finding in the pericardium. Again, this is frequently asymptomatic but pericardial chest pain and effusions may occur. Myocardial involvement is less common but nodules can cause a myocarditis and varying degrees of heart block.

Ocular complications. The most common ocular complication of RA is keratoconjunctivitis sicca, or dry eyes (xerophthalmia). This is usually a consequence of secondary Sjögren's syndrome, and may be associated with dry mouth (xerostomia) and vaginal dryness, the latter leading to dyspareunia. The diagnosis is supported by a positive Schirmer's test, in which an absorbent paper wick is placed just inside the lower eyelid to measure tear production. In Sjögren's syndrome, less than 5 mm of the wick becomes wet in 5 minutes. In patients with coexistent xerostomia, biopsy of a lip salivary gland reveals a lymphocytic infiltrate destroying the glandular tissue.

The episclera lies between the sclera and the conjunctiva, and inflammation (episcleritis) presents with redness and irritation of the eye. Clinically there is a nodular or diffuse brownish-red 'blushing' of the episcleral blood vessels. The condition is benign and usually self-limiting. More sinister is the occurrence of scleritis, which is easily distinguishable as an intensely painful inflammation of the sclera itself (Figure 5.4). Again this can be diffuse or nodular but, in contrast to episcleritis, necrosis and thinning of the sclera may occur, ultimately leading to perforation of the globe. In scleromalacia perforans, on the other hand, thinning is often painless and only presents when the blue-black pigment epithelium becomes visible through the affected translucent sclera. Occasionally the sclera perforates, with protrusion of the pigment epithelium.

Similar processes affecting the cornea result in keratitis, which may be acutely painful (acute necrotizing keratitis). A more insidious and less inflammatory process occurs at the periphery of the cornea

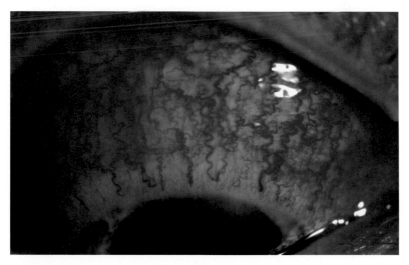

Figure 5.4 Diffuse anterior scleritis. There is marked diffuse injection of the superior globe and a thickened edematous sclera. Clinically this may be intensely painful and tender to light pressure. Image courtesy of Mr W. Innes.

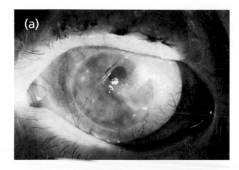

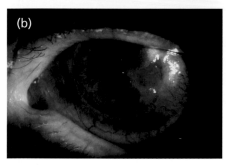

Figure 5.5 Corneal melt.
(a) There is thinning of the lateral aspect of the left cornea, with a surrounding inflammatory infiltrate.
(b) The area of ulceration is highlighted with fluorescein eye drops. Images courtesy of Mr A. Morrell.

(peripheral ulcerative keratitis), resulting in the condition known as 'corneal melt' (Figure 5.5). Destructive processes affecting the sclera and cornea are ophthalmological emergencies, and RA patients should receive regular ophthalmological screening, particularly if they have xerophthalmia, which predisposes to melting.

Skin. Raynaud's symptoms are common in the general population but have an increased prevalence in patients with RA and other connective tissue diseases. The diagnosis requires a triphasic color change during cold exposure. The extremities initially turn white, then blue and ultimately pink from reactive hyperemia. Occasionally the severity of the condition results in digital ulceration and must then be differentiated from cryoglobulinemia and rheumatoid vasculitis.

Rheumatoid vasculitis most commonly affects the small arteries, particularly in the hands and feet, leading to nail-fold infarcts of the fingers and toes (Figure 5.6). Leg ulcers may also be vasculitic in RA (Figure 5.7). More sinister is the involvement of medium-sized arteries, leading to digital gangrene. At this stage multi-organ involvement is

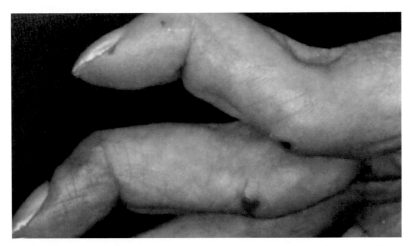

Figure 5.6 A hand displaying the small vasculitic infarcts (and swan neck deformities of the fingers) associated with rheumatoid arthritis.

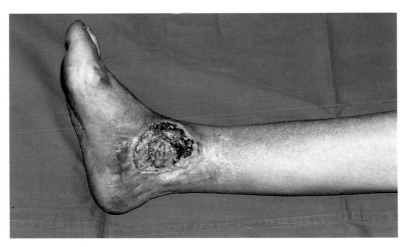

Figure 5.7 A vasculitic leg ulcer in a patient with rheumatoid arthritis. The ulcer has punched-out edges and a necrotic base.

possible, including the mesenteric, coronary or cerebral vessels, although renal involvement is rare.

Osteoporosis is a common and underdiagnosed complication of RA. From disease onset, bone mass decreases for multiple reasons, such as increased bone resorption (see Chapter 3), immobility and

57

glucocorticoid therapy. There are currently few guidelines for the management of low bone mass in RA, but it is important to be aware of risk factors, such as glucocorticoid therapy, and to screen and treat accordingly. In RA, a combination of osteopenia and impaired gait is a recipe for fractures secondary to falls, with a further reduction in mobility and function. (*Fast Facts: Osteoporosis* has more information on this condition.)

Key points – clinical features

- Rheumatoid arthritis (RA) has a variety of articular and extra-articular manifestations.
- The RA spectrum ranges from mild easily controlled disease to progressive destructive disease with organ- and life-threatening extra-articular complications.
- Extra-articular disease activity does not always parallel joint inflammation.
- Patients require close and regular monitoring by a specialist clinician to treat their joint disease and also to promptly diagnose and manage extra-articular manifestations.

Key references

Aletaha D, Neogi T, Silman AJ et al. 2010 Rheumatoid arthritis classification criteria: an American College of Rheumatology/European League Against Rheumatism collaborative initiative. *Arthritis Rheum* 2010;62:2569–81.

Arnett FC, Edworthy SM, Bloch DA et al. The American Rheumatism Association 1987 revised criteria for the classification of rheumatoid arthritis. *Arthritis Rheum* 1988; 31:315–24.

Solomon DH, Curham GC, Rimm E. Cardiovascular risk factors in women with and without rheumatoid arthritis. *Arthritis Rheum* 2004;50:3444–9.

See also those listed on page 12 [Chapter 1].

Initial investigations of inflammatory arthritis (Table 6.1) are guided, on the one hand, by the differential diagnosis (see Table 5.1) and, on the other, by predictors of damage or prognosis (see Chapter 7).

TABLE 6.1

Investigation of recent-onset polyarthritis or polyarthralgia*

Inflammatory markers

- C-reactive protein
- Plasma viscosity
- Erythrocyte sedimentation rate

Hematology

- Full blood count with differential white cell count
- Lupus anticoagulant*

Biochemistry

- Renal function, including urine analysis
- Hepatic function
- Calcium, phosphate
- Uric acid
- Thyroid function tests
- Serum angiotensin-converting enzyme*
- Vitamin D, parathyroid hormone*
- Creatine kinase

Immunology

- ACPA
- Rheumatoid factor
- Anti-nuclear antibody
- Serum immunoglobulins, including electrophoresis
- Anti-neutrophil cytoplasmic antibody*
- Anti-cardiolipin antibody*
- Complement screen*
- Cryoglobulins*
- Tissue typing: HLA-DR, HLA-B27*

Virology/microbiology*

- Parvovirus serology
- Antistreptolysin O titer
- Rubella serology
- Influenza serology
- Mycoplasma serology
- Hepatitis B and C serologies
- HIV serology

CONTINUED

TABLE 6.1 (CONTINUED)

- Yersinia serology
- Campylobacter serology
- Lyme disease serology in endemic areas
- Stool/urethral cultures

Synovial fluid

- To exclude infection
- Positively or negatively birefringent crystals

End-organ investigation

- Radiology of appropriate joints
- HRUS if available
- MRI*
- Chest X-ray*
- Pulmonary function tests*
- Electrocardiogram*
- Echocardiogram*
- Nerve conduction studies/ electromyography*
- Dual X-ray absorptiometry scan*

*Dictated by the clinical picture.
ACPA, anti-citrullinated peptide antibody; HLA, human leukocyte antigen; HRUS, high-resolution ultrasound.

Immunologic investigations

Rheumatoid factor (RF) is an autoantibody with specificity for the Fc region of the immunoglobulin (Ig)G molecule (Figures 6.1 and 3.7). IgM RF is present in up to 75% of RA patients during the course of their disease, although it may be absent at presentation. In contrast, its presence may predate the onset of RA by several years (see page 18). Its precise role in the pathogenesis of RA is unclear, but it is associated with more aggressive disease and extra-articular manifestations. RF is not specific for RA, but may accompany other autoimmune diseases, various acute and chronic infections and certain malignancies (Table 6.2).

The serum titer of RF does not generally correlate with disease activity, except in patients with vasculitis (see page 56), who tend to have a high titer. Conventional tests measure IgM RF, however, whereas some models of RA pathogenesis implicate IgG or IgA RF, which may also be better predictors of long-term prognosis (see

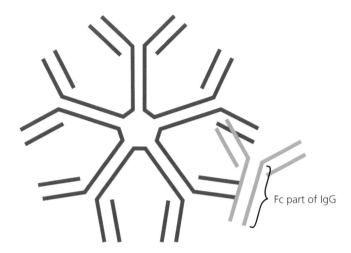

Fc part of IgG

Figure 6.1 Rheumatoid factor (RF) is an autoantibody with specificity for the Fc region of immunoglobulin (Ig)G. Pentameric IgM RF, as shown here, is present in up to 75% of patients during the course of rheumatoid arthritis.

Chapter 7). IgG and IgA RF may, therefore, be more informative but are difficult to measure reliably and tests are not routinely available. Occasionally, an RF is present in serum that precipitates at low temperatures. This is detectable as a cryoglobulin and may be associated with vasculitis and severe Raynaud's phenomenon.

Unlike RF, autoantibodies directed at peptides containing the amino acid citrulline are highly specific for RA (≥ 95%). They may also be present many years before symptomatic onset of RA (see Chapter 2), ultimately appearing in a similar proportion of patients as RF. Citrullinated epitopes are found in many peptides and proteins and are formed by the post-translational deimination of arginyl residues by the enzyme peptidyl arginine deiminase (PADI). Autoantibodies recognizing these epitopes are named anti-citrullinated peptide antibodies (ACPAs), and recognize targets that are potential RA autoantigens, such as citrullinated filaggrin, fibrin, fibrinogen, collagen, alpha-enolase and vimentin. The identification of the ACPA targets that are most closely associated with RA is an area of active

61

TABLE 6.2

Possible causes of positive rheumatoid factor

Infection

- Acute infection (e.g. infectious mononucleosis)
- Chronic bacterial infection (e.g. subacute bacterial endocarditis, tuberculosis, leprosy)
- Parasitic infections (e.g. malaria, schistosomiasis)
- Vaccination

Inflammatory disease

- Rheumatoid arthritis
- Connective tissue diseases (e.g. systemic lupus erythematosus, Sjögren's syndrome)
- Interstitial lung disease
- Chronic active hepatitis
- Cryoglobulinemia

Malignancy

- Lymphoma
- Leukemia
- Myeloma
- Solid tumors

Health

- A positive rheumatoid factor at low titer is common in the normal population

research because this should provide clues to etiology and pathogenesis. Several commercial assays are now available for ACPA detection, most of which use second-generation cyclic citrullinated peptide mixtures (CCP2) as the substrate. The relationship between smoking, the shared epitope and the production of ACPA reflects an important gene–environment interaction in the etiology of RA (see Chapter 2).

ACPA and IgM RF are highly associated with each other, particularly in early RA where over two-thirds of ACPA-positive patients are also positive for IgM RF. As with RF the presence of ACPA, particularly when present at high titer, is associated with more aggressive RA.

Other autoantibodies may also be present in patients with RA. Anti-nuclear antibodies are present in approximately 40% of RA patients, usually at low titer, and have minimal diagnostic or prognostic value. Anti-neutrophil cytoplasmic antibodies (ANCA, usually perinuclear staining [p-]ANCA with specificity for lactoferrin), have been reported in up to 50% of RA patients in some studies. A potential association with more aggressive disease or vasculitis requires confirmation.

Radiology

X-rays are often normal in RA at presentation, or may just show soft-tissue swelling and periarticular osteoporosis around affected joints. Subsequently, classic juxta-articular erosions provide more robust diagnostic information (Figure 6.2). In later disease, erosions spread to the subchondral areas, joint-space narrowing occurs and ultimately subluxation, secondary osteoarthritis and even bony ankylosis may ensue. The rate of development of these changes varies greatly between patients and depends both on therapy and the aggressiveness of the underlying disease. Earliest changes are usually seen in the hands or feet, and X-rays of the hands, wrists and feet are usually performed at presentation. If changes are present these are important prognostically (Chapter 7) but may also help in the differential diagnosis from, for example, inflammatory osteoarthritis, psoriatic arthritis and gout.

In contrast to conventional X-rays, high-resolution ultrasound (HRUS) and MRI may show significant abnormalities in the patient with a very recent onset of joint symptoms. Both modalities continue to be validated as diagnostic tools. MRI detects the water content of tissues, and readily demonstrates articular and periarticular structures (Figure 6.3). Additionally, MRI can capture structural information in several planes, and computer-generated three-dimensional

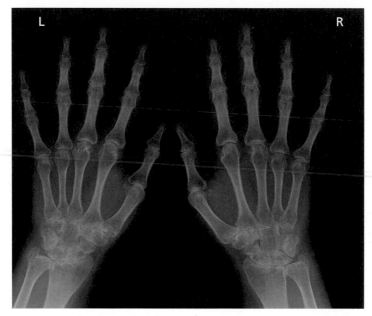

Figure 6.2 Hand radiographs of a patient with erosive rheumatoid arthritis. There is periarticular osteoporosis throughout, with erosions and loss of joint space affecting the carpus, the radiocarpal joints, the thumb bases and several metacarpophalangeal and proximal interphalangeal joints.

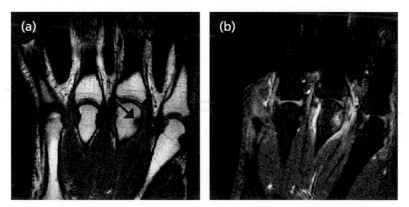

Figure 6.3 Coronal magnetic resonance image of the metacarpophalangeal joints in early rheumatoid arthritis. (a) A T1-weighted image that illustrates a bony erosion (arrow). (b) Corresponding bone edema, as well as adjacent synovial inflammation, is shown on a T2-weighted fat-suppressed image. Images courtesy of Professor P. Conaghan.

reconstructions are possible. In the patient with early RA, inflamed synovium appears as a high signal on T2-weighted fat-suppressed images, and enhances further with the paramagnetic contrast agent gadolinium-DTPA. Bone marrow edema adjacent to the joint surface is a very early abnormality and appears to presage erosion development.

A major disadvantage of MRI is the cost of the equipment and individual scans. It is also a relatively lengthy procedure, requiring the patient to lie still for a considerable period of time in a semi-enclosed space. This may be physically difficult, and some patients also find the procedure claustrophobic, although newer magnet designs are addressing some of these issues. For example, smaller MRI magnets are now available for the study of peripheral joints, providing high-resolution images in an office setting. MRI is the investigation of choice for imaging the rheumatoid cervical spine, however, where it provides high-resolution images of the spinal canal and cord. Similarly, osteonecrosis (avascular necrosis) is readily diagnosed using MRI, for example at the hip. This can occur as a complication of the RA disease process or secondary to therapy with corticosteroids.

HRUS is becoming an increasingly popular rheumatologic imaging technology. It is a relatively inexpensive investigation following initial investments in equipment and training. As with conventional ultrasound, HRUS depends on the relative absorption and reflection of ultrasonic waves by adjacent tissues. In early RA, it is possible to detect small joint effusions and subclinical synovitis. In addition, bone cortical defects are detectable in patients without X-ray erosions. Contemporaneous Power Doppler examination provides information on local blood flow, an important corollary of inflammation (Figure 6.4). HRUS is also useful for imaging tendons and soft tissues, for example in the hands or at the shoulder or ankle where symptoms may be secondary to arthritis, bursitis, tendinitis or fasciitis (see Figure 6.4). Furthermore, ultrasound can be used to guide the placement of injections. This may improve accuracy compared with conventional 'blind' injections, and also permits injections into joints that lack reliable bony landmarks, such as the hip. Rheumatologists themselves are now becoming trained in the use of HRUS, which is

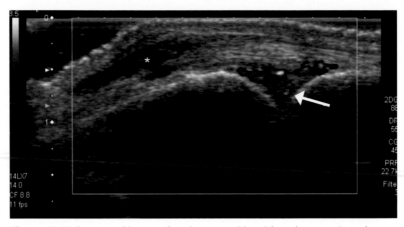

Figure 6.4 Ultrasound image showing synovitis with red power Doppler signal within the metacarpophalangeal joint (arrow), and tenosynovitis (loss of definition, red Doppler signal) in the overlying extensor tendon (asterisk). Image courtesy of Dr P. Platt.

therefore becoming an office, clinic room or bedside aid to the diagnosis, assessment and management of joint disease.

Synovial fluid

Synovial fluid examination is not helpful for the diagnosis of RA. Joint aspiration and microbiological examination is imperative, however, if superadded infection is suspected. This is not uncommon, particularly in the RA patient taking immunosuppressive or biological drugs, and requires prompt diagnosis and treatment. Infection may present as disproportionate inflammation in one or more joints, with or without systemic symptoms, and patients themselves may feel that a distinct process is present in the affected joint. Gout or pseudogout are alternative possibilities, also diagnosed by synovial fluid examination. It is important to appreciate that the macroscopic appearance of synovial fluid is not a reliable guide to the underlying diagnosis. Fluid from acutely inflamed joints secondary to gout or pseudogout may be thick and purulent, whereas fluid from an infected RA joint may appear only slightly cloudy. The definitive diagnosis of these conditions requires Gram stain, crystal analysis using polarized light, and culture of the synovial fluid.

Monitoring RA

In established RA, investigations are aimed at determining disease activity, documenting damage and monitoring drug therapy. A normochromic normocytic anemia suggests poorly controlled disease, as does a low serum albumin. There is no indication to repeat RF titers or ACPA in a seropositive patient, because they do not necessarily correlate with disease activity, but a seronegative patient may convert to seropositivity during the course of their illness. Any patient with poorly controlled disease, particularly if taking glucocorticoid therapy, should be considered for osteoporosis screening by dual emission X-ray absorptiometry (DEXA) or an alternative modality. It is reasonable to repeat radiology of involved joints every 1–2 years to document stabilization or progression of joint damage. Other radiological investigations should be guided by the clinical picture. For example, HRUS is increasingly used to document the presence or absence of synovitis in some cases of established RA where the clinical picture is complicated by a second condition, such as fibromyalgia. The assessment of ongoing RA is discussed in more detail in Chapter 7.

Key points – investigation

- In the acute setting the investigation of polyarthritis is guided primarily by the differential diagnosis.
- There are no pathognomonic tests for rheumatoid arthritis (RA), and investigations may be completely normal at presentation.
- Anti-citrullinated peptide antibodies (ACPAs) are highly specific for RA and have a sensitivity of up to 75%.
- Conventional X-rays may provide diagnostic information but are less sensitive than MRI and high-resolution ultrasound (HRUS), although MRI and HRUS continue to be validated.
- In the chronic setting, investigations are useful for determining disease activity, monitoring therapy and documenting and monitoring joint damage.

Key references

Brown AK. Using ultrasonography to facilitate best practice in diagnosis and management of RA. *Nat Rev Rheumatol* 2009;5:698–706.

Cheung PP, Dougados M, Gossec L. Reliability of ultrasonography to detect synovitis in rheumatoid arthritis: a systematic literature review of 35 studies (1,415 patients). *Arthritis Care Res (Hoboken)* 2010;62:323–34.

Freeston JE, Bird P, Conaghan PG. The role of MRI in rheumatoid arthritis: research and clinical issues. *Curr Opin Rheumatol* 2009;21:95–101.

Nishimura K, Sugiyama D, Kogata Y et al. Meta-analysis: diagnostic accuracy of anti-cyclic citrullinated peptide antibody and rheumatoid factor for rheumatoid arthritis. *Ann Intern Med* 2007;146:797–808.

When a patient develops rheumatoid arthritis (RA), they are keen
to understand their long-term outlook. RA can still result in severe
disability and a dependent existence, but increasingly effective
drugs and management strategies have improved the outlook for the
majority of patients. Furthermore, mild disease can be readily
controlled with relatively non-toxic drugs or may even spontaneously
remit. It is not possible to provide a completely accurate picture
for each patient, but a number of prognostic factors have now been
defined. It is also important to gauge accurately the current status
of a patient, in order to decide on the need for, and effectiveness of,
therapy, and to draw valid conclusions when new and existing
therapies are compared.

Prognosis

There are two aspects of RA prognosis to consider. First, which
patients with inflammatory synovitis of recent onset will develop
chronic and progressive, as opposed to mild and self-limiting, disease?
Second, of the former group, which factors predict more severe joint
damage? With regard to the first question, recent studies suggest that
inflammation of the metacarpophalangeal (MCP) joints lasting for
longer than 12 weeks is the simplest predictor of chronicity, and
symptoms that resolve before this time tend not to recur. At present
there is no single laboratory marker that can provide equivalent
information at an earlier time point. The 2010 American College
of Rheumatology (ACR)/European League Against Rheumatism
(EULAR) criteria have been developed to help predict the development
of chronic and damaging synovitis in individuals with recent-onset
inflammatory arthritis (see Chapter 5).

Factors that are associated with more severe damage are listed in
Table 7.1. These include simple demographic factors such as female
sex, an older age at disease onset and a lower formal educational level,
each of which imparts a worse prognosis. Smoking is also associated

TABLE 7.1

Factors associated with a poor prognosis in rheumatoid arthritis

- Female sex
- Older age at disease onset
- Longer disease duration at presentation
- Low formal educational level
- Smoker
- Poor functional status at presentation
- Positive ACPA
- Positive RF
- Raised acute-phase response at presentation
- Shared-epitope-positive HLA type
- Reduced ability to oxidize sulfur (low sulfoxidation status)
- X-ray-evident joint damage at presentation

ACPA, anti-citrullinated peptide antibody; HLA, human leukocyte antigen; RF, rheumatoid factor.

with more erosive disease, potentially via its association with anti-citrullinated peptide antibody (ACPA) positivity. At presentation, a longer duration of symptoms, functional limitation (see below), or a raised acute-phase response are all associated with a worse prognosis. Adverse immunogenetic features include seropositivity for RF and/or ACPA, a tissue type that includes human leukocyte antigen (HLA) genes encoding the shared epitope (strongly associated with ACPA positivity), or a reduced capacity to oxidize sulfur (sulfoxidation status). Lastly, the presence of X-ray erosions at presentation is, not surprisingly, a poor-prognostic sign.

Patients who are seen in academic referral centers are likely to have more severe disease and usually possess more of the above-mentioned features associated with poor prognosis. On the other hand, certain subtypes of RA, such as polymyalgic onset at an advanced age, appear to have a more favorable prognosis.

Assessment of ongoing RA

The assessment of RA is both objective and subjective. For example, a swollen-joint count and a measure of the acute-phase response provide useful objective measures. On the other hand, entirely subjective features, such as fatiguability or the duration of early-morning joint stiffness, may be more important from the patient's perspective. Additionally, satisfaction with medical management may depend more upon the patient's functional capabilities. These will encompass personal (washing, dressing, preparing a meal), social (e.g. ability to leave the house and attend a party) and economic (ability to remain in their current employment in a full-time capacity) activities. Importantly, the same physical impairment can result in varying degrees of disability. Thus, a deformity affecting the non-dominant hand will be of more consequence to a musician than to a writer. Furthermore, the same deformity in an elderly person may prevent them from dressing themselves and therefore could be socially isolating. Psychological factors, including coping strategies and illness perception, are also important determinants of disability, as are social perspectives. Thus, the elderly person living alone will be more disabled than if they have a partner to help them dress. Anxiety and depression also have major impacts on the degree of disability experienced.

Assessing function. Functional impairment may be evident at presentation. At this stage of the disease, it usually reflects the degree of joint inflammation, although later the cumulative effects of damage to tendons, ligaments, cartilage and bone contribute more (Figure 7.1). A number of self-completion questionnaires that focus on function and participation have been designed and validated. Some are condition-specific, such as the Stanford Health Assessment Questionnaire (HAQ) or the Arthritis Impact Measurement Scale (AIMS), whereas others are generic, such as the short form 36 (SF36). These questionnaires collect information along a number of dimensions (e.g. self-care, hand function, mobility, work and play) that relate to the activities of daily living and psychosocial functioning (Figure 7.2). They are useful tools for assessing current disease status

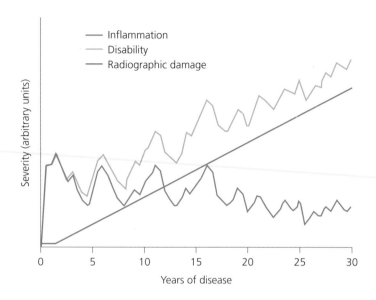

Figure 7.1 Theoretical model of contributors to functional impairment in rheumatoid arthritis. Reproduced with permission from Kirwan, 2001.

but also carry prognostic significance (see above). Some instruments, such as the modified HAQ (mHAQ), specifically seek changes in function since the previous assessment, via 'transitional' questions. Others, such as the McMaster Toronto Arthritis (MACTAR) Patient Preference Questionnaire, adopt a patient-specific perspective, and attempt to measure personal handicap. Thus, the patient nominates specific roles pertinent to their personal situation and, at each assessment, rates their ability to fulfill those roles.

A simple alternative to questionnaires is to observe and measure patients completing simple tasks such as walking a set distance, fastening and unfastening buttons, or by assessing grip strength using an inflatable cuff. Patients can also be allocated to specific 'functional classes' (Table 7.2), but these are relatively insensitive to short-term change.

Quality of life (QoL) encompasses a number of dimensions, including physical, social, psychological and economic aspects. Functional

Please tick the ONE best answer for your abilities

At this moment, you are able to:	Without any difficulty	With some difficulty	With much difficulty	Unable to do
Dress yourself, including tying shoelaces and fastening buttons?				
Get in or out of bed?				
Lift a full cup or glass to your mouth?				
Walk outdoors on flat ground?				
Wash and dry your entire body?				
Bend down to pick up clothing from the floor?				
Turn normal taps on or off?				
Get in and out of a car?				

Figure 7.2 Example of a self-assessment functional questionnaire for patients. Reproduced with permission from Pincus et al., 1989.

TABLE 7.2

American College of Rheumatology functional classification of rheumatoid arthritis

Class I: Completely able to perform usual activities of daily living (self-care, vocational and avocational)

Class II: Able to perform usual self-care and vocational activities, but limited in avocational activities

Class III: Able to perform usual self-care activities, but limited in vocational and avocational activities

Class IV: Limited in ability to perform usual self-care, vocational and avocational activities

Usual self-care includes dressing, feeding, bathing, grooming and toileting. Vocational (work, school, homemaking) and avocational (recreational and/or leisure) activities are patient-desired and age- and sex-specific.
Reproduced with permission from Hochberg et al., 1992.

capabilities are an important determinant of QoL, and some questionnaires address both. Generic examples include the Nottingham Health Profile and the SF36, whereas the rheumatoid arthritis QoL (RAQoL) instrument was designed specifically for patients with RA.

Composite scores. RA is a complex disease and cannot be assessed using a single measure. Therefore, in accordance with the variable manifestations and outcomes of RA, composite assessment criteria have been devised, although debate continues regarding the 'minimal data set' needed to provide a reliable picture of the individual patient. The ACR response criteria were designed for assessing outcomes in the clinical trials setting. These measure changes from baseline in the number of tender and swollen joints, acute-phase response, a functional measure (e.g. HAQ score), visual analog scale for pain, and global assessment of disease by patient and physician, also on a visual analog scale. A 20% improvement in swollen and tender joint counts, and in three of the remaining five parameters, represents an ACR20 response. This is the minimum required for efficacy in most trials. ACR50 and ACR70 responses are calculated in a similar fashion.

While useful for monitoring clinical trials, these scores have not been validated in the routine clinical setting. Furthermore, they relate to a particular baseline, and a given improvement may be more difficult to achieve from a less active baseline. Thus, a 20% improvement from a baseline of five swollen joints may be more difficult to achieve than from a baseline of 20 swollen joints. In contrast, the disease activity score (DAS; Table 7.3) provides a continuous variable which does not require reference to a baseline. The DAS is a complex measure that was derived by studying a number of disease activity criteria in patients with variable disease activity, and applying assorted statistical measures, including discriminant analysis and multiple regression analysis. Because of its continuous nature, a patient can be assigned a meaningful DAS at any stage of their disease, and inter-patient comparisons can also be made. Increasingly, the DAS is being used in the routine clinic setting. It provides a longitudinal quantitative measure of RA activity by which to judge the effectiveness of current management and the need for adjustment. In the clinical trial setting, improvement targets can be defined as both a reduction in DAS and also a target level of DAS, providing for good, moderate and nil improvements. The DAS28 is a modification based on 28 swollen and tender joints (see Table 7.3).

Alternatives to the DAS include the simplified disease activity index (SDAI) and the clinical disease activity index (CDAI). The former is a simple numerical sum of joint counts, patient and clinician global assessments and C-reactive protein (CRP); the latter removes CRP from the calculation, providing a 'bedside' composite score. An increasing emphasis is now being placed on patient-reported outcome measures (PROMs) to synergize with, or sometimes replace, these composite scores. Fatigue and sleep disturbance, as just two examples, are poorly captured by conventional outcome measures such as DAS28 and yet are some of the most disabling symptoms to patients. The Routine Assessment of Patient Index Data 3 (RAPID3) or Multi Dimensional Health Assessment Questionnaire (MDHAQ) is a patient-completed composite score that incorporates physical function, pain and patient global assessment that is simple to perform. Many patients can also reliably perform their own joint counts, providing further self-assessment information.

TABLE 7.3

Disease activity score (DAS) and DAS28

$$DAS = 0.53938 \sqrt{(RAI)} + 0.06465(S44) + 0.330(lnESR) + 0.00722(GH)$$
$$DAS28 = 0.56 \sqrt{(T28)} + 0.28 \sqrt{(S28)} + 0.70(lnESR) + 0.014(GH)$$

DAS28, DAS including the 28-joint count; GH, patient's assessment of general health in millimeters on a visual analog scale of 100 mm; lnESR, natural logarithm of erythrocyte sedimentation rate; RAI, Ritchie Articular Index, a graded joint tenderness score based on 53 joints; S28, ungraded joint swelling count based on 28 joints; S44, ungraded joint swelling count based on | 44 joints; T28, ungraded joint tenderness count based on 28 joints.
From Van der Heijde et al., 1993 and Van Gestel et al., 1998.

Radiology. Functional impairment in chronic RA is influenced by the amount of joint damage (see Figure 7.1). This can be assessed using conventional X-rays, according to a number of semi-quantitative grading systems such as the Larsen and Sharp scores. In essence, these quantify radiographic change in a number of prespecified joints of the hands (and the feet in the modified Sharp score) to provide a single score. The Sharp score considers erosions and joint-space narrowing independently, and can also be used to discriminate between new joints affected versus progression in previously affected joints. The rate of progression and severity of joint damage are both relevant to functional impairment.

X-ray damage usually occurs slowly and changes are rarely visible on images taken a few months apart. Thus, although a gold standard for structural outcome, radiology is of limited use in early disease or for monitoring the effects of therapy in the short term. Furthermore, Larsen and Sharp scores are seldom recorded in routine clinical practice, as opposed to the research setting. In contrast, high-resolution ultrasound (HRUS) and MRI can detect changes in synovitis and bone marrow edema over periods of weeks to months (see Chapter 6), and may become valuable adjuncts for the monitoring and assessment of RA.

Biochemical markers of damage. Quantifiable markers of tissue destruction should provide a complementary and dynamic adjunct to radiological monitoring as the complex biochemistry of synovium, bone and cartilage is elucidated and tissue-specific markers defined. For example, serum osteocalcin levels provide a dynamic measure of osteoblastic activity, and serum and urine levels of type I collagen c-telopeptide (CTX-I) reflect bone resorption. Urinary deoxypyridinolone cross-links may also reflect bone damage. Cartilage breakdown releases type II collagen fragments such as cross-linked C-terminal telopeptides (CTX-II) and type II collagen helical peptide (Helix II), and matrix proteins such as cartilage oligomeric protein (COMP), also quantifiable in serum or urine. Markers of collagen synthesis have also been identified but no consistently useful assays are yet available for measuring proteoglycan synthesis or breakdown.

Other potential markers of tissue damage include circulating matrix metalloproteinase (MMP) levels, particularly MMP3 levels. Some of these assays are starting to provide useful information in the clinical trial setting, when applied to groups of patients receiving different treatments. Currently, however, none has sufficient sensitivity or specificity to be applied routinely in the clinic to provide an index of tissue damage for the individual patient.

Remission

Remission is the ultimate aim of RA therapy and is defined according to strict criteria, established in 1982 by Pinals et al. (Table 7.4). These criteria are very exacting, however, and are unlikely to be fulfilled by patients with joint damage. At the time of press replacement criteria were being developed jointly by ACR and EULAR. The SDAI and CDAI also have very stringent remission criteria. DAS remission is defined by a DAS $\leq$ 1.6 or DAS28 $\leq$ 2.6 but neither include all possible joints – in particular, DAS28 ignores the feet. A DAS28 $\leq$ 3.2 defines low disease activity. Alternative criteria are being defined and debated, including the use of synovial imaging. Thus, synovitis may be

---

TABLE 7.4

American College of Rheumatology criteria for clinical remission* of rheumatoid arthritis

A minimum of five of the following for at least 2 consecutive months:

- Morning stiffness not exceeding 15 minutes

- No fatigue

- No joint pain

- No joint tenderness or pain on motion

- No soft-tissue swelling in joints or tendon sheaths

- ESR < 30 mm/hour (females) or < 20 mm/hour (males)

*Clinical remission cannot be diagnosed in the presence of manifestations of active vasculitis, pericarditis, pleuritis, myositis, and/or unexplained recent weight loss or fever. ESR, erythrocyte sedimentation rate.
Adapted from Pinals et al., 1982.

present on MRI or HRUS in the absence of clinically detectable inflammation, and may underlie the progression of joint damage in some patients during apparent clinical 'remission'. Prospective studies have identified a number of predictors of remission including male sex, short interval between symptom onset and diagnosis, and lack of circulating autoantibodies. The adoption of 'treatment-to-target' strategies in the management of RA (see Chapter 8) will result in an increasing emphasis in clinical practice on achievement of remission and low disease activity states.

Key points – assessment

- Rheumatoid arthritis can be assessed using objective clinical scores such as swollen-joint counts, biochemical and radiological parameters such as acute-phase response and joint X-rays, and subjective measures of pain, function and participation.
- Most information is captured in composite scores such as the disease activity score (DAS).
- Quality of life is of overriding importance to the patient, and should always be considered during routine assessments.
- A number of patient-reported outcome measures (PROMs) are being developed that quantify symptoms such as fatigue and sleep.

Key references

Aletaha D, Smolen JS. The Simplified Disease Activity Index and Clinical Disease Activity Index to monitor patients in standard clinical care. *Rheum Dis Clin North Am* 2009;35:759–72.

Hochberg MC, Chang RW, Dwosh I et al. The American College of Rheumatology 1991 revised criteria for the classification of global functional status in rheumatoid arthritis. *Arthritis Rheum* 1992;35: 498–502.

Katchamart W, Johnson S, Lin HJ et al. Predictors for remission in rheumatoid arthritis patients: a systematic review. *Arthritis Care Res (Hoboken)* 2010;62:1128–43.

Kirwan JR. Links between radiologic change, disability, and pathology in rheumatoid arthritis. *J Rheumatol* 2001;28:881–6.

Pinals RS, Baum J, Bland J et al. Preliminary criteria for clinical remission in rheumatoid arthritis. *Bull Rheum Dis* 1982;32:7–10.

Pincus T, Callahan LF, Brooks RH et al. Self-report questionnaire scores in rheumatoid arthritis compared with traditional physical, radiographic, and laboratory measures. *Ann Intern Med* 1989;110:259–66.

Pincus T, Swearingen CJ, Bergman MJ et al. RAPID3 (Routine Assessment of Patient Index Data) on an MDHAQ (Multidimensional Health Assessment Questionnaire): agreement with DAS28 (Disease Activity Score) and CDAI (Clinical Disease Activity Index) activity categories, scored in five versus more than ninety seconds. *Arthritis Care Res (Hoboken)* 2010;62:181–9.

Skapenko A, Prots I, Schulze-Koops H. Prognostic factors in rheumatoid arthritis in the era of biologic agents. *Nat Rev Rheumatol* 2009;5:491–6.

Syversen SW, Haavardsholm EA, Boyesen P et al. Biomarkers in early rheumatoid arthritis: longitudinal associations with inflammation and joint destruction measured by magnetic resonance imaging and conventional radiographs. *Ann Rheum Dis* 2010;69:845–50.

van der Heijde DM, van 't Hof M, van Riel PL, van de Putte LB. Development of a disease activity score based on judgment in clinical practice by rheumatologists. *J Rheumatol* 1993;20:579–81.

van der Helm-van Mil AH, le Cessie S, van Dongen H et al. A prediction rule for disease outcome in patients with recent-onset undifferentiated arthritis: how to guide individual treatment decisions. *Arthritis Rheum* 2007;56:433–40.

van Gestel AM, Haagsma CJ, van Riel PL. Validation of rheumatoid arthritis improvement criteria that include simplified joint counts. *Arthritis Rheum* 1998;41:1845–50.

The acute and chronic consequences of rheumatoid arthritis (RA) result from persistent, misdirected and inadequately controlled inflammation that causes tissue destruction and loss of function. Consequently, management strategies for RA have become highly refined over the past 10 years. The concept of long-term therapy with non-steroidal anti-inflammatory drugs (NSAIDs) or corticosteroids while awaiting a natural remission is no longer acceptable. Rheumatologists today initiate disease-modifying antirheumatic drug (DMARD) therapy as soon as the diagnosis of RA is secure. Subsequently, therapy is aggressively adjusted until a state of low disease activity or remission is achieved. For this reason, it is critical that patients are referred for specialist assessment as soon as the diagnosis of RA is suspected, and even before the results of investigations are available. Early control of inflammation and the disease process is essential to minimize irreversible joint damage and functional disability. Most patients will commence therapy with methotrexate, either alone or ideally in combination with other DMARDs. With aggressive DMARD therapy a proportion of patients will achieve disease remission, and those who do not can now receive biological therapies (see Chapter 9) within a few months of diagnosis.

The patient must be fully educated about treatment options and expectations from the outset, and decisions regarding drug therapy must be mutually agreed. Furthermore, the rheumatologist must serve as an advocate for the patient with regard to treatment and drug monitoring programs. In the USA this is particularly important, in light of potential restrictions due to changes in the healthcare reimbursement system and managed care. Economic considerations have also become important in the UK, although recent guidelines from the National Institute for Health and Clinical Excellence (NICE) have reduced some previous restrictions on the prescribing of biologics (see Chapter 9).

Patients treated by rheumatologists have a slower rate of disease progression, and less joint damage and disability, than those not receiving care from an arthritis specialist. The expertise of the rheumatologist is in advising drug regimens, referring to rehabilitation specialists, and recognizing the importance and timing of orthopedic consultation and procedures.

Non-pharmacological approaches

Reduction of joint stress can be accomplished by local rest of an inflamed joint. Weight reduction, splinting, use of walking aids and specially designed utensils can all significantly reduce stress on joints. During significant disease flares, vigorous activity should be avoided, although full range of motion of joints should be maintained by a graded exercise program to prevent contractures and muscular atrophy.

The role of physical and occupational therapy, podiatry, nursing educational programs and vocational rehabilitation cannot be overemphasized. Rest, splinting of involved joints, adaptive equipment, appropriate exercise programs, orthotics, foot care and bespoke shoes, and nutritional and physiological support are all essential ingredients of a successful treatment regimen.

Pharmacological approaches – overview

The traditional 'pyramid' approach to the treatment of RA was to begin with symptomatic treatment of inflammation using NSAIDs in addition to rest and corticosteroid injections. If the disease did not significantly improve with these simple treatments, then more potent DMARDs were added. It is now clear, however, that effective therapy early in the course of RA results in a long-term reduction in joint damage compared to delayed therapy, the so-called window of opportunity. This has led to the general principle that inflammation should be controlled as completely and as soon as possible by the early and aggressive introduction of DMARDs. The currently approved non-biological drugs for treating RA are listed in Table 8.1. Most of these require monitoring for the prompt detection of potential adverse effects, although the precise monitoring recommendations vary from center to center. The British Society for Rheumatology, the European League Against Rheumatism and the American College of

TABLE 8.1

Non-biological drugs used in rheumatoid arthritis

- Non-steroidal anti-inflammatory drugs (COX-non-selective and COX2-selective)
- Analgesics
- Corticosteroids
  - Systemic (oral or parenteral)
  - Intra-articular
- Disease-modifying antirheumatic drugs
  - Methotrexate
  - Antimalarials: hydroxychloroquine, chloroquine
  - Sulfasalazine
  - Gold salts
  - Leflunomide
  - Ciclosporin (cyclosporin[e] A)
  - D-penicillamine
  - Azathioprine
  - Cyclophosphamide

COX, cyclooxygenase.

Rheumatology have each developed guidelines for the use and monitoring of RA therapies.

Non-steroidal anti-inflammatory drugs

NSAIDs remain one of the most frequently prescribed class of drugs in the treatment of patients with RA, at least early in the disease process. The major effect of these agents is to reduce joint pain and improve joint function. There is no evidence that NSAIDs have any effect on the underlying disease process, however, and exacerbation of symptoms occurs quickly after metabolic elimination of the drugs. They are rarely, if ever, treatment for RA in isolation and without DMARD therapy.

The major therapeutic effect of NSAIDs relates to their ability to suppress the synthesis of prostaglandins by inhibiting the enzyme cyclooxygenase (COX). COX exists in two isoforms: COX-1 and COX-2. COX-1 is expressed constitutively in many tissues and is primarily responsible for the production of prostaglandins by vascular endothelium, platelets and gastric mucosa, leading to hemostatic and cytoprotective effects. It is also important for the regulation of renal blood flow. COX-2 is undetectable in most normal tissues; its expression increases during development of inflammation and can be induced by several pro-inflammatory stimuli.

Both traditional non-specific NSAIDs as well as more selective COX-2 inhibitors are approved for use in RA. The principal benefit of COX-2 inhibitors is the production of analgesic and anti-inflammatory effects comparable with those of the non-selective NSAIDs, but with lower risk of serious gastrointestinal adverse reactions and without prolongation of the bleeding time. Renal side effects may still occur, however, as a result of constitutive COX-2 expression in the kidney. Furthermore, data regarding the potential adverse cardiovascular consequences of both non-selective and COX-2 specific drugs has resulted in a significant reduction in their chronic use. In the UK, in recent guidance, NICE has revised its recommendations on the use of these drugs, recommending their use at the lowest effective dose for the shortest possible period of time (Table 8.2).

Corticosteroids

Corticosteroids have a long history in the treatment of many rheumatic diseases and they are still a key element in the management of RA. They produce rapid and potent suppression of inflammation, with improvement in fatigue, joint pain and swelling. Prednisone (prednisolone) is most frequently used for RA at a dose of 5–10 mg once daily to minimize adrenal suppression and metabolic side effects. Therapy is often initiated in patients with active disease while awaiting the full therapeutic effect of DMARDs. Recent clinical trials have confirmed the ability of corticosteroids to rapidly control inflammation in patients with recent-onset RA when used in combination with DMARD therapy. In these trials, tapering and

TABLE 8.2

The management of symptom control in adults, from NICE Clinical Guideline 79 (2009)

- Offer analgesics (for example, paracetamol, codeine or compound analgesics) if pain control is not adequate, to potentially reduce the need for long-term treatment with NSAIDs or COX-2 inhibitors

- Oral NSAIDs/COX-2 inhibitors should be used at the lowest effective dose for the shortest possible period of time

- When offering an oral NSAID/COX-2 inhibitor, the first choice should be either a standard NSAID or a COX-2 inhibitor. In either case, these should be co-prescribed with a PPI, choosing the one with the lowest acquisition cost

- All oral NSAIDs/COX-2 inhibitors have analgesic effects of a similar magnitude but vary in their potential gastrointestinal, liver and cardiorenal toxicity; therefore, when choosing the agent and dose, take into account individual patient risk factors, including age. When prescribing consider appropriate assessment and/or ongoing monitoring of these risk factors

- If a person needs to take low-dose aspirin, consider other analgesics before substituting or adding an NSAID or COX-2 inhibitor (with a PPI) if pain relief is ineffective or insufficient

- If NSAIDs or COX-2 inhibitors are not providing satisfactory symptom control, review the disease-modifying or biological drug regimen

COX, cyclooxygenase; NICE, National Institute for Health and Clinical Excellence; NSAID, non-steroidal anti-inflammatory drug; PPI, proton pump inhibitor.

cessation is generally accomplished in 3–6 months. In contrast, corticosteroid therapy can be difficult to discontinue in established RA, and tapering should be gradual to avoid disease flares: e.g. 0.5–1.0 mg/day every few weeks to months. For this reason some rheumatologists prefer to use a single parenteral dose of a depot steroid preparation (e.g. methylprednisolone acetate or triamcinolone acetonide) when rapid control of inflammation is required. This can be administered by intramuscular injection, with efficacy lasting for

6–8 weeks. Intra-articular steroid injections are particularly useful for controlling, with minimal systemic effects, a local flare in joints that show disproportionate involvement.

Adverse effects. The adverse effects of corticosteroids limit their long-term use, especially in high doses. Careful surveillance and preventive interventions are needed to avoid undesired complications. Periodic assessment for steroid-induced osteoporosis has become a standard of care for patients receiving chronic corticosteroid therapy, and patients should undergo regular bone densitometry to assess fracture risk. The greatest risk of bone loss occurs during the first 6–12 months of corticosteroid use. If bone densitometry is not readily available, most rheumatologists recommend prophylactic treatment, for example with a bisphosphonate, in any patient starting prednisone treatment and who is likely to receive a dose of 7.5 mg per day or higher for at least 6 months. In addition, the immunosuppressive consequences of chronic corticosteroid use should not be underestimated, even at doses of less than 10 mg per day.

Notwithstanding the above, the use of corticosteroids displays significant geographic variation. In the UK, NICE recommends long-term corticosteroid use in established RA only after their potential complications have been fully discussed with the patient and all other treatment options, including biologics, have been offered.

Disease-modifying antirheumatic drugs

All patients with RA are candidates for DMARD therapy, initiated at the time of diagnosis. DMARDs lack an analgesic effect, and can take weeks to months to provide clinical benefit. When used as monotherapy they may only moderate the disease process, without completely suppressing inflammation. Therefore, they are increasingly used in combination with one another. The Dutch Behandel Stratagieen (BeSt) study compared various strategies for DMARD use in early RA and concluded that combination therapy of methotrexate, sulfasalazine and hydroxychloroquine, with a tapered dose of prednisone, was as effective as infliximab (see Chapter 9) plus methotrexate. By rapidly controlling inflammation, both were superior

85

to sequential DMARD monotherapy, or 'step-up' therapy, where failure of one DMARD led to the addition of a second, and so on.

Several studies have shown that a very important aspect of DMARD use is regular patient assessment (e.g. with a disease activity score including the 28-joint count [DAS28]), and adjustment of therapy if a target level of disease activity has not been achieved (usually low disease activity, DAS28 ≤ 3.2; or remission, DAS28 ≤ 2.6), so-called 'treating to target'. This includes the use of systemic or intra-articular steroids when required. In this way inflammation is effectively suppressed, regardless of the drugs used to achieve it, with minimization of joint damage. It may be possible to taper one or more elements of a combination regimen once disease is in clinical remission (step-down therapy). NICE guidance for the management of early RA is shown in Table 8.3.

Antimalarials (chloroquine and hydroxychloroquine) are commonly used drugs with a favorable toxicity–benefit profile. Chloroquine is more popular in mainland Europe and appears to be more potent but more toxic than hydroxychloroquine, which is used in the USA and UK. Hydroxychloroquine (200–400 mg daily) is often used in early mild disease and as background therapy when another DMARD is started. There are no data available to prove that hydroxychloroquine alone reduces or prevents radiological damage from RA. The most serious potential adverse event is ocular toxicity secondary to retinal deposits, particularly with chloroquine. This is extremely rare with hydroxychloroquine, but it is recommended that patients undergo an ophthalmology examination before starting therapy and at intervals thereafter.

Methotrexate has become the most commonly used DMARD for RA as a result of its favorable efficacy/toxicity profile and low cost. More than 50% of patients taking methotrexate continue the drug for more than 5 years, which is longer than for any other DMARD. Despite its effectiveness, the precise mechanism of action of methotrexate in RA remains uncertain. Many rheumatologists prescribe parenteral (subcutaneous or intramuscular) methotrexate following ineffective

TABLE 8.3

The management of early rheumatoid arthritis, from NICE Clinical Guideline 79 (2009)

- In people with newly diagnosed active RA, offer a combination of DMARDs (including methotrexate and at least one other DMARD, plus short-term glucocorticoids) as first-line treatment as soon as possible, ideally within 3 months of the onset of persistent symptoms

- Consider offering short-term treatment with glucocorticoids (oral, intramuscular or intra-articular) to rapidly improve symptoms in people with newly diagnosed RA if they are not already receiving glucocorticoids as part of DMARD combination therapy

- In people with recent-onset RA receiving combination DMARD therapy and in whom sustained and satisfactory levels of disease control have been achieved, cautiously try to reduce drug doses to levels that still maintain disease control

- In people with newly diagnosed RA for whom combination DMARD therapy is not appropriate start DMARD monotherapy, placing greater emphasis on fast escalation to a clinically effective dose rather than on the choice of DMARD

DMARD, disease-modifying antirheumatic drug; NICE, National Institute for Health and Clinical Excellence; RA, rheumatoid arthritis.

oral therapy because this drug has variable absorption when taken by mouth, and the parenteral route is less likely to cause nausea. Unfortunately, plasma level testing is not reliable or routinely available. The usual dose ranges from 15 to 25 mg once weekly. It is essential that the patient understands that dosing is weekly and not daily, as the latter will result in potentially fatal bone marrow suppression.

Contraindications and monitoring. Use of methotrexate in patients with renal insufficiency or on dialysis should be avoided. Guidelines for monitoring patients with RA while on methotrexate have been established by a number of bodies. Baseline tests for all patients prior to initiation of therapy should include a complete blood count (CBC), serum creatinine and liver function tests (LFTs), and chest X-ray.

Hepatitis B and C serologies are recommended in the USA, and some rheumatologists also perform pulmonary function testing routinely. Hematological monitoring and LFTs (transaminases, alkaline phosphatase) should subsequently be performed on a regular basis. Men and women of childbearing age must be made aware that methotrexate is teratogenic; they should practice effective birth control during use and for at least 6 months after the drug has been discontinued.

Side effects. Nausea, mouth ulcers, bone marrow suppression and hepatocellular injury are the main side effects. Less common complications include interstitial pneumonitis, rarely pulmonary fibrosis, and occasionally opportunistic infections. Gastrointestinal symptoms may be avoided by the concomitant use of folic acid (5 mg once weekly or 1 mg once daily) or a change to parenteral administration. Folic acid may also reduce hepatic enzyme abnormalities associated with methotrexate use.

Sulfasalazine is a conjugate of a salicylate and a sulfapyridine molecule. The usual dose is 1.0–1.5 g twice daily. In addition to the anti-inflammatory effect of the salicylate component, sulfasalazine appears to have immunomodulatory effects, and has an efficacy similar to that of methotrexate. It is frequently used in combination with other DMARDs.

Side effects. Gastrointestinal symptoms are the most common side effects, and are often resolved with dose reduction. Hematological consequences include aplastic anemia, agranulocytosis and hemolytic anemia, and CBC monitoring is recommended on a regular basis, in addition to LFTs.

Leflunomide is a further DMARD with immunomodulatory properties. It is an isoxazole prodrug that is rapidly converted in the gastrointestinal tract to an active metabolite following oral administration. The active metabolite binds to and reversibly inhibits the enzyme dihydroorate dehydrogenase (DHODH), the rate-limiting enzyme in de novo pyrimidine synthesis, which is essential for lymphocyte turnover. Leflunomide therefore has inhibitory effects on lymphocyte proliferation. It slows radiographic damage in RA to a similar degree as methotrexate and sulfasalazine. It takes about 7–8 weeks for this drug to reach steady-state levels in the blood and a loading dose of 100 mg/day for 3 days may be used, followed by a maintenance dose of 10–20 mg/day.

Side effects. Adverse events include bone marrow toxicity, reversible alopecia, skin rash, stomatitis, diarrhea, hypertension and elevation in liver enzymes. Routine monitoring of CBC, LFTs and blood pressure are required. Leflunomide is also teratogenic. It has an extremely long half-life and, if required, its elimination can be accelerated with cholestyramine or activated charcoal.

Gold compounds, because of their effectiveness in suppressing synovitis, were the most popular disease-modifying agents in the 1970s and early 1980s. However, because of their relative toxicity and the existence of many new alternatives, they are less often used today. The parenteral preparations currently in use are aurothioglucose (Solganal/ Solganol, available in the USA) and sodium aurothiomalate (Myocrisin, available in the UK), administered intramuscularly. An initial test dose of 10 mg should be administered before starting weekly therapy at 50 mg. The dosing interval can be increased once an effect is established. Auranofin, an oral preparation, is less effective than intramuscular gold and rarely used. The mechanism of action of gold salts has not been definitively established, but it is postulated that gold compounds act at many points in the immunoinflammatory pathway.

Side effects. The most common adverse effects of gold are mucocutaneous reactions, including stomatitis, pruritis and various forms of dermatitis. Proteinuria may occur and is usually mild, although rarely reaches the nephrotic range. Leukopenia, thrombocytopenia and aplastic anemia are rare but have potentially fatal consequences. CBC and urinalysis should be performed before each injection.

D-**Penicillamine** is also rarely prescribed today. It has a similar adverse-effect profile to that of gold salts, and side effects occur frequently. When used, it is initiated at a dose of 125–250 mg daily, with slow escalation to a maintenance dose of 500–750 mg daily if tolerated.

Ciclosporin (previously cyclosporin[e] A) is a drug that inhibits T cell function and is a mainstay in preventing rejection of transplanted organs. In RA it is effective as monotherapy and as an adjunct to methotrexate. In general, however, it is reserved for refractory cases of RA, primarily because of its nephrotoxic adverse events which preclude its widespread use.

Cytotoxic drugs, including azathioprine and cyclophosphamide, are generally reserved for patients with refractory RA who have failed conventional therapy. They are little used today in RA, because of their toxicity and existence of new alternatives. Cyclophosphamide, however, is used in patients with rheumatoid vasculitis or organ-threatening extra-articular disease such as interstitial pneumonitis. The usual mode of administration is by intermittent intravenous 'pulses', often accompanied by intravenous corticosteroid.

Surgery

Although modern management strategies are less focused on orthopedic surgery, the benefits of surgery, when required, should not be underestimated. In particular, joint replacements have become the standard of care for large joints (e.g. hip, knee) with end-stage disease and loss of cartilage. In general there are two types of indication for surgery. The first is to deal with irreversibly damaged tissues and specific disease complications. This category includes joint replacements but also, for example, forefoot surgery for intractable pain secondary to rheumatoid deformities. Repair of damaged tendons, for example at the shoulder, also falls under this heading, as would the removal of problematic rheumatoid nodules. The second category includes prophylactic surgery to prevent deformity and loss of function. Synovectomy, for example, is still employed occasionally as a treatment for refractory joint or tendon sheath involvement before the destruction of surrounding tissues ensues. This is of particular clinical relevance at the hand, where flexor tendon involvement is common. Similarly, stabilization of the cervical spine will prevent progressive myelopathy in the predisposed patient (see page 50).

The optimal timing of, and potential benefit to be gained from, orthopedic surgery in the RA patient requires skilled judgment. Similarly, both local and systemic disease activity must be optimally controlled perioperatively. It follows that pre- and postoperative assessment and care requires a multidisciplinary approach involving not only surgeon and rheumatologist, but also occupational therapist and physiotherapist. Most important of all, the patient must be absolutely clear as to the indication for surgery (relief of pain, preservation of function or both) and likely outcome. For example, pain-relieving elbow surgery may improve quality of life but not necessarily upper limb function.

Key points – traditional measures

- Non-steroidal anti-inflammatory drugs (NSAIDs) and corticosteroids provide symptomatic relief but should almost never be used in isolation.
- Disease-modifying antirheumatic drugs (DMARDs) are the mainstay of pharmacological therapy, and their use in early rheumatoid arthritis (RA) reduces long-term irreversible joint damage.
- Treatment-to-target strategies, including combination DMARD therapy, rapidly suppress inflammation and minimize long-term damage and disability.
- DMARDs are generally safe with appropriate monitoring, but adverse events are potentially life-threatening if missed.
- Optimal therapy also includes access to allied health professionals such as nurse specialists, physiotherapists, occupational therapists and podiatrists.
- The need for, and timing of, surgery requires skilled judgment.
- Consequently, the patient with RA is optimally managed from disease onset by a rheumatologist and their multidisciplinary team.

Key references

Boers M, Verhoeven AC, Markusse HM et al. Randomised comparison of combined step-down prednisolone, methotrexate and sulphasalazine with sulphasalazine alone in early rheumatoid arthritis. *Lancet* 1997;350:309–18.

Goekoop-Ruiterman YP, de Vries-Bouwstra JK, Allaart CF et al. Clinical and radiographic outcomes of four different treatment strategies in patients with early rheumatoid arthritis (the BeSt study): a randomized, controlled trial. *Arthritis Rheum* 2005;52:3381–90.

Grigor C, Capell H, Stirling A et al. Effect of a treatment strategy of tight control for rheumatoid arthritis (the TICORA study): a single-blind randomised controlled trial. *Lancet* 2004;364:263–9.

Kearney PM, Baigent C, Godwin J et al. Do selective cyclo-oxygenase-2 inhibitors and traditional non-steroidal anti-inflammatory drugs increase the risk of atherothrombosis? Meta-analysis of randomised trials. *BMJ* 2006; 332:1302–8.

Landewe RB, Boers M, Verhoeven AC et al. COBRA combination therapy in patients with early rheumatoid arthritis: long-term structural benefits of a brief intervention. *Arthritis Rheum* 2002;46:347–56.

Mottonen T, Hannonen P, Leirisalo-Repo M et al. Comparison of combination therapy with single-drug therapy in early rheumatoid arthritis: a randomised trial. FIN-RACo trial group. *Lancet* 1999;353:1568–73.

National Institute for Health and Clinical Excellence. *The Management of Rheumatoid Arthritis in Adults (Clinical Guideline 79)*. London: NICE, 2009. Available from www.nice.org.uk/CG79, last accessed 5 October 2010.

Rantalaiho V, Korpela M, Hannonen P et al. The good initial response to therapy with a combination of traditional disease-modifying antirheumatic drugs is sustained over time: the eleven-year results of the Finnish rheumatoid arthritis combination therapy trial. *Arthritis Rheum* 2009;60:1222–31.

van der Kooij SM, Goekoop-Ruiterman YP, de Vries-Bouwstra JK et al. Drug-free remission, functioning and radiographic damage after 4 years of response-driven treatment in patients with recent-onset rheumatoid arthritis. *Ann Rheum Dis* 2009;68:914–21.

Advances in translational research have led to a better understanding of the pathogenesis of rheumatoid arthritis (RA). Combined with advances in biotechnology, this has led to the development of several biological therapies for RA. Biological therapies are produced from living cells rather than by chemical synthesis and, generally, are monoclonal antibodies (mAbs) or soluble derivatives of cell surface receptors. Those used to treat RA target specific molecules or receptors in the immune and/or inflammatory process (Table 9.1). Depending on their precise molecular structure mAbs can be chimeric (murine variable [V]-region, human constant [C]-region); humanized (human in sequence apart from murine complementarity determining regions); or fully human (derived from human B cells or gene libraries, or from transgenic mice with human immunoglobulin genes).

TABLE 9.1

Biological therapies approved for treating rheumatoid arthritis

TNF antagonists

- Adalimumab
- Certolizumab pegol
- Etanercept
- Golimumab
- Infliximab

IL-1 antagonist

- Anakinra

IL-6 antagonist

- Tocilizumab

B-cell-depleting mAb

- Rituximab

Co-stimulation blocker

- Abatacept

IL, interleukin; mAb, monoclonal antibody; TNF, tumor necrosis factor.
Note: mAbs of chimeric (mouse/human) structure have the suffix –ximab; humanized mAbs have the suffix –zumab; fully human mAbs have the suffix –mumab; soluble receptors have the suffix –cept.

In the UK, the National Institute for Health and Clinical Excellence (NICE) has issued extensive guidance on the use of biological agents to treat RA. This states that tumor necrosis factor (TNF) antagonists (see Table 9.1) can be prescribed to patients who have not responded adequately to at least two disease-modifying antirheumatic drugs (DMARDs), including methotrexate (unless contraindicated), and have a disease activity score 28 (DAS28) greater than 5.1 (high disease activity) on two occasions 1 month apart. Methotrexate should be co-prescribed with TNF inhibitors unless there is a contraindication. Patients who develop side effects during the first 3 months may switch to a second anti-TNF agent, but otherwise rituximab (in combination with methotrexate, see pages 98–100) should be prescribed after anti-TNF failure. If there is a contraindication to rituximab, or side effects develop, a second anti-TNF, abatacept (see page 100) or tocilizumab (see pages 101–2) may be prescribed. In addition, tocilizumab is recommended for patients who respond inadequately to rituximab. Biologics should only be prescribed by a consultant rheumatologist with monitoring of the DAS28 as a measure of effectiveness. NICE guidance states that anti-TNF therapy should only be continued if the DAS28 falls by at least 1.2 units after 6 months of therapy. At present in the USA the use of biological therapies is reserved for patients who have had an incomplete or inadequate response to DMARDs such as methotrexate.

Tumor necrosis factor antagonists

The development of drugs that target TNF has been an enormous advance. In the last 12 years, the US Food and Drug Administration (FDA) and the European Medicines Agency (EMA) have both approved five TNF antagonists for the treatment of RA: etanercept, infliximab, adalimumab, golimumab and certolizumab pegol (Figure 9.1).

The transmembrane precursor of soluble TNF is found on a variety of cells throughout the body. Macrophages appear to be the primary source of active TNF in RA, via TNF converting enzyme (TACE)-mediated cleavage of transmembrane TNF. After being shed from the cell surface, TNF molecules aggregate into trimolecular complexes

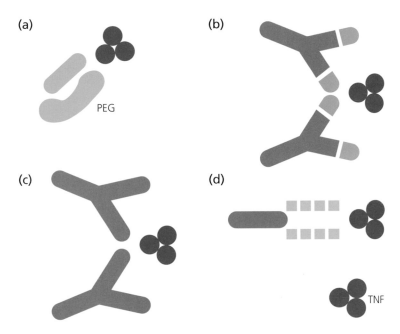

Figure 9.1 Therapies that block tumor necrosis factor (TNF): (a) certolizumab pegol; (b) infliximab; (c) adalimumab, golimumab; and (d) etanercept. PEG, polyethylene glycol.

that subsequently bind receptors on a variety of cells, including fibroblasts, leukocytes and endothelial cells. Two TNF receptors have been described: the p55 (type I) receptor and the p75 (type II) receptor. TACE also cleaves the extracellular domain of the cell surface TNF receptors, forming soluble TNF receptors (sTNFRs). These circulating sTNFRs are then free to bind the trimolecular TNF complexes, rendering them biologically inactive; thus, the sTNFRs function as natural inhibitors of TNF-mediated inflammation.

A variety of physiological functions have been ascribed to TNF–TNF-receptor interactions. TNF blocks the action of lipoprotein lipase, causing severe cachexia in experimental models of chronic infection. Additionally, TNF induces programmed cell death (apoptosis) and stimulates the release of several other pro-inflammatory cytokines, including interleukin (IL)-1, IL-6 and IL-8. It also induces the release of matrix metalloproteinases (MMPs) from fibroblasts, chondrocytes and neutrophils, activates osteoclasts, and upregulates the expression of endothelial adhesion molecules, leading to the migration of leukocytes into extravascular tissues.

Etanercept is a genetically engineered molecule containing two human p75 TNF receptor extracellular domains linked to the Fc portion of human immunoglobulin (Ig)G1. The recommended dosage for adults is 50 mg by subcutaneous injection weekly, or 25 mg twice weekly.

Infliximab is a chimeric anti-TNF mAb, administered by intravenous infusion. Co-administration of methotrexate with infliximab significantly reduces the formation of antibodies directed against the murine portion of the molecule (antiglobulins), which can otherwise neutralize its effectiveness. Infliximab is currently recommended for use only with concomitant methotrexate therapy, at a dose of 3 mg/kg every 8 weeks, following three 'loading' infusions at weeks 0, 2 and 6.

Adalimumab is a humanized mAb against TNF. It is administered by subcutaneous injection every 2 weeks.

Most recently, golimumab and certolizumab pegol have received regulatory approval for treating RA. Golimumab is a fully human mAb. Certolizumab pegol differs from the other TNF antagonists in being a humanized 'fragment antigen binding' (Fab') attached to polyethylene glycol (PEG), which increases its half-life.

These five TNF inhibitors show excellent effectiveness in both early and established RA. In addition to improvements in inflammation and joint damage, patients receiving TNF inhibitors also report important reductions in fatigue and malaise with significant quality-of-life benefits. Aside from differences in immunogenicity, half-life and route of administration, there are theoretical differences between the five TNF inhibitors. For example, etanercept also neutralizes lymphotoxin, although the contribution of this feature to effectiveness or toxicity is uncertain.

Patients who may benefit. Not all RA patients respond to TNF antagonists and, at present, there are no factors that reliably predict effectiveness. Currently these drugs are licensed for use in patients who have failed one or more conventional DMARD (the precise license depends on geographic location). Their effectiveness approximates inversely with the duration of RA – thus they are more effective in early disease and least effective in very late disease.

Adverse effects. Postmarketing surveillance has led to the recognition of certain adverse effects of TNF blockade. These include reactivation of tuberculosis, resulting in atypical clinical presentations such as disseminated disease and a lack of classic caseating granulomas on histology. Appropriate screening (history, chest X-ray and purified protein derivative [PPD] skin testing or stimulated interferon-γ release assays) is mandatory prior to beginning any anti-TNF agent. RA patients overall are at higher risk for serious infections than healthy peers. According to some (but not all) registry data, anti-TNF agents may further increase the risk, particularly with regard to skin and soft tissue, bone and joint, lung and opportunistic infections.

Other adverse events from anti-TNF therapies include local injection-site reactions (with subcutaneously administered agents) and systemic infusion reactions with infliximab, which may relate to the development of neutralizing antiglobulins and be associated with loss of effect. Other probable drug-related events include induction of autoantibodies (e.g. antinuclear antibodies [ANA], anti double-stranded DNA antibodies), drug-induced lupus, drug-induced vasculitis, demyelination, congestive heart failure and worsening of interstitial lung disease. Despite initial concerns there is, as yet, no evidence that anti-TNF agents increase the risk of malignancy or lymphoma in RA patients, with the possible exception of non-melanoma skin cancers.

Interleukin-1 antagonism

IL-1 is thought to play a major pro-inflammatory role in RA, but also to be an important stimulus to erosion development and bone destruction. IL-1 receptor antagonist (IL-1ra) and soluble IL-1 receptors (sIL-1Rs) are natural inhibitors of IL-1 and are produced locally at sites of inflammation. In RA, however, there appears to be an imbalance that favors the pro-inflammatory actions of IL-1.

97

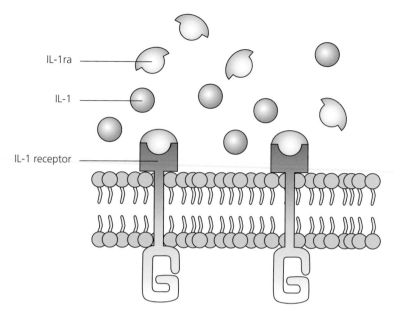

IL-1ra

IL-1

IL-1 receptor

Figure 9.2 Interleukin-1 (IL-1) receptor antagonist (IL-1ra) blocks binding of IL-1α and IL-1β to the IL-1 type I receptor.

Anakinra is a recombinant form of IL-1ra, which is licensed for the treatment of RA and designed to shift the balance back toward an anti-inflammatory state (Figure 9.2). It is generally well tolerated. Mild transient injection-site reactions are the commonest reported adverse events. Overall, its effectiveness is less than TNF antagonists and other biological therapies. In the UK, NICE has not approved its use to treat RA.

B cell depletion

Not only are B cells the precursors of autoantibody-producing plasma cells but they are also efficient antigen-presenting cells (APCs), and additionally produce cytokines such as TNF, IL-6 and lymphotoxin (Figure 9.3). Proof of the central role of B cells in RA pathogenesis has come from a novel therapeutic approach. Rituximab is a chimeric mAb specific for CD20, a phosphoprotein expressed on the surface of mature and naive B cells but absent from B cell precursors and plasma cells. Rituximab depletes circulating B cells and produces therapeutic

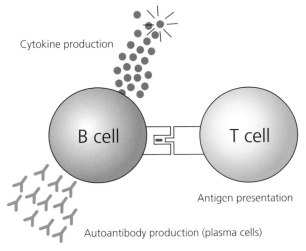

Figure 9.3 Functions of B cells relevant to rheumatoid arthritis. In addition to being the precursors of antibody-producing plasma cells, B cells also secrete cytokines and present antigen to T cells.

benefit in RA similar to that achieved with TNF antagonists. It is approved for treatment of RA patients for whom anti-TNF therapy has failed. Rituximab is administered intravenously on two separate occasions, usually 2 weeks apart. The licensed dose is 1000 mg at the first and second infusions, each infusion preceded by 100 mg i.v. methylprednisolone to reduce the incidence of infusion reactions (see below). Repeated courses of rituximab may be administered if symptoms return after an initial improvement with rituximab, usually about 6 months later. Emerging data suggest that rituximab is more effective in RA patients with circulating autoantibodies (rheumatoid factor [RF] and/or anti-citrullinated peptide antibodies [ACPA]).

Infusion reactions are the most frequent adverse events reported with rituximab, affecting up to 30% of patients. They are most common with the first dose of the first course of therapy and are probably secondary to cytokine release associated with B cell lysis. Common symptoms include fever, chills and urticaria, which can progress to angioedema and bronchospasm, though this is rare. No new safety signals have been noted from the use of rituximab in RA when compared with the extensive data available from its use in oncology (more than 1 million patients treated for non-Hodgkin's lymphoma and chronic lymphocytic leukemia). No increased risk of infections or opportunistic infections has been noted in RA patients, even after multiple courses of therapy, although there is a cumulative reduction in Ig levels, particularly IgM, with repeated cycles of therapy. Recent reports of progressive multifocal leucoencephalopathy in a small number of patients receiving rituximab for RA remain unexplained, although the majority of the patients were receiving or had received additional immunosuppression.

Co-stimulation blockade

In addition to interaction of the T cell receptor with its peptide-MHC ligand, a succession of secondary, or co-stimulatory, molecular interactions are required for full T cell activation. The main second signal is provided by interaction of CD28 on the T cell with B7.1 (CD80) and B7.2 (CD86) on the APC. Following activation, cytotoxic T-lymphocyte-associated protein 4 (CTLA4 [also known as CD152]) is upregulated on the T cell. This is a downregulatory molecule that has a 100-fold higher affinity for CD80 and CD86 than does CD28, and contributes to the cessation of the immune response.

Abatacept is the first approved biological therapy that alters T cell function by blocking co-stimulatory pathways between APCs and T cells. It comprises the extracellular domain of CTLA4 fused to the Fc of human IgG_1, which has been modified to avoid target cell lysis. By competing with CD28 for binding to CD80 and CD86, abatacept downregulates T cell activation. Clinical trials have demonstrated abatacept to be effective in RA patients with early disease as well as in disease refractory to methotrexate and TNF blockade. It is administered intravenously every 4 weeks following three 'loading' infusions at weeks 0, 2 and 4. Abatacept is generally well tolerated with a slightly increased risk of upper respiratory tract infections. Based on available data there does not appear to be an increased risk of opportunistic infections or malignancies.

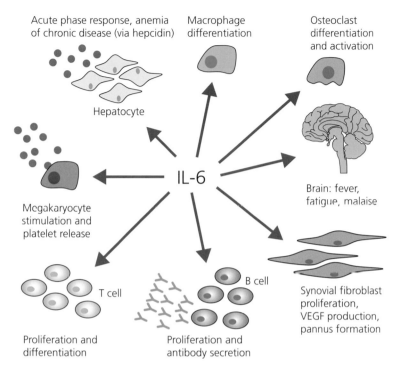

Figure 9.4 Functions of interleukin-6 (IL-6) relevant to rheumatoid arthritis. VEGF, vascular endothelial growth factor.

Interleukin-6 receptor blockade

IL-6 plays a key role in the pathogenesis of RA (Figure 9.4). It stimulates B and T cells and, via vascular endothelial growth factor (VEGF) production, leads to new blood vessel development. Alongside stimulatory effects on synovial fibroblasts, this leads to pannus formation. IL-6 also stimulates megakaryocytes, leading to thrombocytosis, and hepatocytes to produce acute phase proteins. It also activates osteoclast precursors leading to bone resorption, and has important systemic effects including malaise, fatigue, fever and anemia of chronic disease via hepcidin production.

Tocilizumab is a humanized anti IL-6 receptor (Il-6R) mAb that neutralizes the effects of IL-6. Its licensed dose is 8 mg/kg every 4 weeks by intravenous infusion. Several phase III trials have demonstrated clinical efficacy in RA patients at all disease stages, from early disease to anti-TNF failure.

As IL-6 plays a key role in immune surveillance, its inhibition might be expected to be associated with an increased risk of infections. The controlled trials suggest a possible slight increase in bacterial infections, similar to other biological therapies. However, suppression of the acute phase response by tocilizumab may mask warning signs of infection. Other adverse events include transient neutropenia, transient elevation in liver enzymes and an increase in lipid levels. These events are usually mild and reversible and occur at a low frequency. There is no evidence for enhanced vascular events in patients receiving tocilizumab, although this is an area of continuing research with several biological therapies.

The research agenda

Biological therapies have provided a major boost to our therapeutic options in RA, but there remains a significant research agenda surrounding their use. For example, all biological therapies can be immunogenic, provoking the development of potentially neutralizing antiglobulins in some, but not all, recipients. Understanding factors that predispose to immunogenicity should result in improved outcomes of therapy as well as a better appreciation of the incidence and clinical significance of antiglobulins.

Understanding why some patients do not respond to biological therapies remains a major challenge and provides opportunities for further dissection of the pathogenic mechanisms operative in RA. Factors predisposing to opportunistic or unusual infections also require clarification. Finally, the costs of these potent therapies will need to be evaluated in terms of their long-term benefit, with particular regard to work stability, the predicted reduction in joint replacements, and their potential to provide improved quality of life and lifespan (see Chapter 4). The question whether they should replace methotrexate or sulfasalazine as the DMARDs of first choice will be answered only as the use of these agents increases.

Now that we have nine biological therapies approved to treat RA, our major challenge over the next several years will be directed towards how to best use these in individual patients. Specifically, we need to develop biomarkers of the immune abnormalities in each patient so we can apply the most appropriate treatment (personalized medicine). In addition, we will need more research as to how to use these newer therapies in combination with more traditional medications such as methotrexate.

Key points – biological therapies

- Nine biological therapies are now licensed for the treatment of RA. These block cytokines or their receptors (tumor necrosis factor [TNF], interleukin [IL]-1 and IL-6), deplete B cells or interfere with T cell activation.
- Biologics are expensive drugs, produced from living cells, that require parenteral (intravenous or subcutaneous) administration. They slow joint damage more effectively than traditional disease-modifying antirheumatic drugs.
- Patients vary in their response to biologics, presumably reflecting important inter-patient differences in disease pathogenesis and drug pharmacokinetics.
- Prolonged experience will be required to provide a true therapeutic ratio and an accurate economic evaluation of these drugs.
- A major research agenda relates to how to target these drugs to the patients who will derive most benefit from them (personalized medicine).

Key references

Isaacs JD. Antibody engineering to develop new antirheumatic therapies. *Arthritis Res Ther* 2009;11:225.

Isaacs JD. Therapeutic agents for patients with rheumatoid arthritis and an inadequate response to tumour necrosis factor-alpha antagonists. *Expert Opin Biol Ther* 2009;9:1463–75.

Moots RJ, Ostor AJ, Isaacs JD. Will treatment of rheumatoid arthritis with an IL-6R inhibitor help facilitate the 'age of remission'? *Expert Opin Investig Drugs* 2009;18:1687–99.

Nam JL, Winthrop KL, van Vollenhoven RF et al. Current evidence for the management of rheumatoid arthritis with biological disease-modifying antirheumatic drugs: a systematic literature review informing the EULAR recommendations for the management of RA. *Ann Rheum Dis* 2010;69:976–86.

National Institute for Health and Clinical Excellence. *The Management of Rheumatoid Arthritis in Adults (Clinical Guideline 79)*. London: NICE, 2009. Available from www.nice.org.uk/CG79, last accessed 5 October 2010.

National Institute for Health and Clinical Excellence. *Adalimumab, Etanercept and Infliximab for the Treatment of Rheumatoid Arthritis (NICE Technology Appraisal 130)*. London: NICE, 2007. Available from www.nice.org.uk/TA130, last accessed 5 October 2010.

National Institute for Health and Clinical Excellence. *Adalimumab, Etanercept, Infliximab, Rituximab and Abatacept for the Treatment of Rheumatoid Arthritis after the Failure of a TNF Inhibitor (NICE Technology Appraisal 195)*. London: NICE, 2010. Available from www.nice.org.uk/TA195, last accessed 5 October 2010.

National Institute for Health and Clinical Excellence. *Tocilizumab for the Treatment of Rheumatoid Arthritis (NICE Technology Appraisal 198)*. London: NICE, 2010. Available from www.nice.org.uk/TA198, last accessed 5 October 2010.

Strand V, Kimberly R, Isaacs JD. Biologic therapies in rheumatology: lessons learned, future directions. *Nat Rev Drug Discov* 2007;6:75–92.

Taylor PC. Pharmacology of TNF blockade in rheumatoid arthritis and other chronic inflammatory diseases. *Curr Opin Pharmacol* 2010;10: 308–15.

Numerous novel potential targets for biological as well as oral therapies are currently under investigation. Those that are showing the most promise are outlined below.

Interleukin (IL)-1 Trap and monoclonal antibody to IL-1

A 'Trap' is a cytokine inhibitor that uses different high-affinity receptor components to bind the target ligand. A molecule targeting IL-1 ('IL-1 Trap') comprises the extracellular domains of both IL-1 receptor components (type I receptor and receptor accessory protein) linked to the Fc portion of human immunoglobulin (Ig)G_1. This recombinant molecule (rilonacept) binds to IL-1α and IL-1β and blocks interaction with the IL-1 receptor (Figure 10.1). A monoclonal antibody (mAb) to IL-1 (canakinumab) is also being tested as a therapy for several inflammatory and autoimmune diseases.

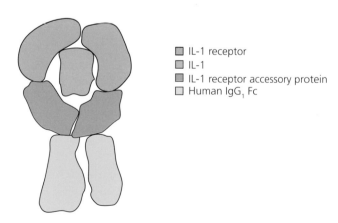

■ IL-1 receptor
■ IL-1
■ IL-1 receptor accessory protein
□ Human IgG$_1$ Fc

Figure 10.1 Interleukin-1 (IL-1) is trapped within the IL-1 Trap (rilonacept) and unable to associate with the endogenous IL-1 receptor. IgG$_1$, immunoglobulin G$_1$.

Interleukin-17

IL-17, first described in 1995, is an attractive target in rheumatoid arthritis (RA), though it has been less studied than many of the previously described cytokines. It is produced by T helper 17 (TH17) cells, which are physiologically important for fighting extracellular bacterial infections, but which are also found at the site of inflammation in a number of autoimmune states. It has pro-inflammatory activity and may be important early in the inflammatory response (see also Chapter 3). It activates endothelial cells, promoting leukocyte recruitment and activation, and also induces a variety of other inflammatory mediators, including tumor necrosis factor (TNF), IL-1, IL-6 and IL-8. IL-17 may have direct catabolic properties in cartilage through upregulation of nitric oxide production from chondrocytes. It also has important effects on bone, promoting osteoclastic bone resorption. Clinical trials of anti-IL-17 mAbs will determine whether IL-17 inhibition will be as effective as other cytokine inhibitors.

Signal transmission inhibition

Inflammatory and destructive responses require appropriate gene activation. In turn, these genes are activated through cascades of signaling molecules.

Janus kinase inhibitors. The Janus kinase (JAK) family of tyrosine kinases (TYKs) comprises JAK1, JAK2, JAK3 and TYK2. All family members are expressed ubiquitously except for JAK3, which is expressed exclusively in leukocytes. JAK3 associates with the common γ-chain, which is a component of the IL-2 receptor as well as other cytokine receptors (including IL-4, IL-7, IL-9, IL-15 and IL-21). JAK3 plays a crucial role in regulating leukocyte function, becoming activated following IL-2 binding to the IL-2 receptor. Once activated, JAK3 phosphorylates specific tyrosine residues on the receptor, leading to the recruitment of specific signal transducers and activators of transcription (STATs). The STATs are then phosphorylated and reorient as dimers; they are released from the receptor and translocate to the nucleus where they act as powerful regulators of gene transcription. Clinical trials of JAK inhibitors in patients with RA have yielded encouraging results, both from efficacy and toxicity standpoints. These are chemically synthesized orally bioavailable drugs, which provides a potential advantage over biological therapies. Phase III trials are in progress.

Spleen tyrosine kinase inhibitors. Spleen tyrosine kinase (SYK), an intracellular tyrosine kinase, is a key mediator of Fcγ receptor, B cell receptor and toll-like receptor signaling. All three of these pathways are of potential pathogenic significance in RA and an orally bioavailable SYK inhibitor is being studied in RA, with encouraging results to date.

Gene therapy

Some of the biological therapies, such as IL-1 receptor antagonist (IL-1ra), are limited by an extremely short half-life. Gene therapy provides a potential means of overcoming the requirement for daily injections. Essentially, the gene encoding the therapeutic product is inserted into a non-replicative viral vector. This is then used to introduce the gene into a recipient either systemically via the bloodstream, or locally into tissues. A number of examples have been successfully applied to animal models of arthritis. The main limitations at present are generalized safety issues relating to the use of viral vectors, and the need to identify robust methods for regulating transcription and translation of the therapeutic gene.

Therapeutic tolerance

Therapeutic tolerance refers to methods of switching off unwanted immune responses, usually by targeting the T cell–antigen-presenting cell (APC) interaction. In animal models, therapeutic tolerance has been possible for many years, allowing organ graft transplantation without immune suppression, and effectively providing a cure for autoimmunity. Translation to the clinic has been slow, but over recent years there have been major advances both in the application of tolerogenic therapies, and in their monitoring. For example, the use of non-activating anti-CD3 mAbs in patients with recent-onset type 1 diabetes has effectively delayed disease progression for up to 4 years.

A number of cellular therapies are also being developed as potential tolerogenic agents. These include purified and expanded regulatory T cells, tolerogenic dendritic cells and mesenchymal stem cells which, in addition to their tissue engineering potential (see below), also have powerful immunomodulatory properties.

Stem cell biology

Mesenchymal stem cells (MSCs) are the precursors of osteoblasts, chondrocytes, myocytes and adipocytes. Rapid advances are being made in the isolation, expansion and culture of these cells, which could result in the generation of 'replacement parts' for joints in the laboratory. The main challenges are identifying optimal growth factors and conditions, and methods to guide the ultimate structure of laboratory-grown tissues, including the use of artificial scaffolds. Although such technology is likely to be applied initially to osteoarthritic joints, a role in RA may become evident, particularly if mesenchymal defects are shown to play a primary role in disease pathogenesis.

Pre-RA

Chapter 2 (page 18) highlighted that circulating autoantibodies appear many years before the onset of RA symptoms. Imaging studies have also indicated that synovitis can be present in joints for weeks to months before symptoms occur. Clinical trials of many therapies have demonstrated optimal results in early disease and attention is starting to turn to the preclinical phase of RA for two reasons. First, the likelihood of switching off disease and obtaining long-term remission, for example using tolerogenic therapies (see above), appears much higher before disease becomes established. Second, if it were possible to identify individuals with a high likelihood of developing RA, it may be possible to institute preventive measures. These could reflect lifestyle changes, such as smoking cessation or weight loss, or even mild therapeutic interventions such as hydroxychloroquine or a brief course of corticosteroids. Susceptible individuals might be identified either by screening family members for autoantibodies and tissue type, or even population screening for similar factors. A number of social and ethical issues need to be addressed before the adoption of such strategies, even in the trial setting, but this is an area of intense current interest.

Epigenetics

The sequencing of the human genome has led to huge advances in understanding the genetics of diseases such as RA (see Chapter 2). It is now evident, however, that DNA sequence is only one determinant of an individual's phenotype. Epigenetics is the study of phenotypic and gene-expression changes caused by mechanisms other than changes in the DNA sequence. These include DNA silencing by methylation, and transcriptional modification of genes by histone acetylation. Another important influence comes from microRNAs, which are genome-encoded small RNA molecules that influence the transcription and translation of genes. A number of important epigenetic modifications have been linked to human disease and, importantly, these processes are readily targetable. Aspects of the RA pathogenic process attributable to epigenetic modification have already been modulated in vitro and drugs that target epigenetic processes will soon be developed for RA.

Advances in surgery

Although reconstructive surgery has been one of the major advances for improving the quality of life of many RA patients, there are limitations; these include loosening of the prosthetic joints and inadequate prosthetic replacements for several joints (e.g. ankle, shoulder). A large body of knowledge is accumulating concerning prosthetic joint loosening, which should result in the development of techniques and strategies to prolong the life of artificial joints. Furthermore, progress is being made in the design and implementation of novel joint prostheses.

Key points – therapeutic developments

- A large number of drugs are currently in clinical trials for rheumatoid arthritis (RA); several target novel mediators and pathways, incorporating concepts such as epigenetic modification.
- Signaling pathway inhibitors are orally active drugs with potencies similar to biological therapies. Their successful passage through phase III trials could have a major impact on RA management.
- Mesenchymal stem cells have both immunomodulatory and tissue engineering potential. They could develop into an important cellular therapy for diseases such as RA.
- In the future, rheumatologists may identify and treat patients in the presymptomatic phase of RA, using approaches such as therapeutic tolerance induction.

Key references

Cooles FA, Isaacs JD. Treating to re-establish tolerance in inflammatory arthritis – lessons from other diseases. *Best Pract Res Clin Rheumatol* 2010;24:497–511.

Isaacs JD. The changing face of rheumatoid arthritis: sustained remission for all? *Nat Rev Immunol* 2010;10:605–11.

Jungel A, Ospelt C, Gay S. What can we learn from epigenetics in the year 2009? *Curr Opin Rheumatol* 2010;22:284–92.

Leung PS, Dhirapong A, Wu PY, Tao MH. Gene therapy in autoimmune diseases: challenges and opportunities. *Autoimmun Rev* 2010;9:170–4.

Useful addresses

UK
Arthritis Care
(Patient support group [e-mail
address is for young people with
arthritis])
Tel: +44 (0)20 7380 6500
Helpline: 0808 800 4050
info@arthritiscare.org.uk
www.arthritiscare.org.uk

Arthritis and Musculoskeletal Alliance
(Umbrella body representing a
broad range of interests across
service user, professional and
research groups working in the
field of musculoskeletal conditions)
Tel: +44 (0)20 7842 0910/11
info@arma.uk.net
www.arma.uk.net

Arthritis Research UK
(Charity funding rheumatology
research and patient support)
Tel: +44 (0)300 790 0400
enquiries@arthritisresearchuk.org
www.arthritisresearchuk.org

British Society for Rheumatology
(Rheumatologists' association)
Tel: +44 (0)20 7842 0900
bsr@rheumatology.org.uk
www.rheumatology.org.uk

National Rheumatoid Arthritis Society
(Organization providing support
and information for patients and
health professionals)
Tel: 0845 458 3969/
+44 (0)1628 823524
Helpline: 0800 298 7650
helpline@nras.org.uk
enquiries@nras.org.uk
www.nras.org.uk

Primary Care Rheumatology Society
(General practitioners interested in
rheumatology)
Tel: +44 (0)1609 774794
helen@pcrsociety.org
www.pcrsociety.org

USA
American College of Rheumatology
(Rheumatologists' association)
Tel: +1 404 633 3777
acr@rheumatology.org
www.rheumatology.org

Arthritis Foundation
(Patient support group)
Toll-free: 800 283 7800
www.arthritis.org

International

Arthritis Australia

(Organization providing support
and information for patients and
health professionals)
Tel: +61 (0)2 9518 4441
Toll-free: 1800 111 101
info@arthritisaustralia.com.au
www.arthritisaustralia.com.au

Australian Rheumatology Association

(Rheumatologists' association)
Tel: +61 (0)2 9256 5458/9626
www.rheumatology.org.au

European League Against Rheumatism

(Rheumatologists' association)
Tel: +41 44 716 30 30
eular@eular.org
www.eular.org

International League of Associations for Rheumatology

(Collaboration of organizations
that works to support progress in
the practice and education of
rheumatology in countries where
there is an exceptional need)
www.ilar.org

Index

113

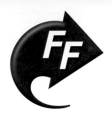

Fast Facts – the ultimate medical handbook series covers 72 topics,
including:

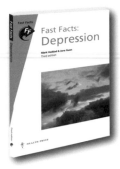

Fast Facts:
Depression

Mark Haddad & Jane Gunn
Third edition

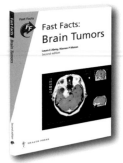

Fast Facts:
Brain Tumors

Laurie E Abrey, Warren P Mason
Second edition

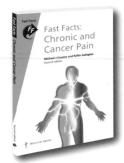

Fast Facts:
Chronic and Cancer Pain

Michael J Cousins and Rollin Gallagher
Second edition

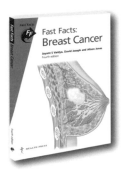

Fast Facts:
Breast Cancer

Jayant S Vaidya, David Joseph and Alison Jones
Fourth edition

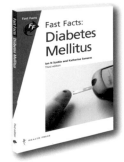

Fast Facts:
Diabetes Mellitus

Ian N Scobie and Katherine Samaras
Third edition

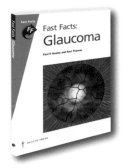

Fast Facts:
Glaucoma

Paul R Healey and Ravi Thomas

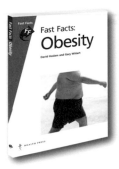

Fast Facts:
Obesity

David Haslam and Gary Wittert

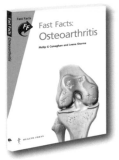

Fast Facts:
Osteoarthritis

Philip G Conaghan and Leena Sharma

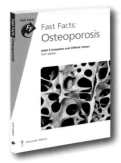

Fast Facts:
Osteoporosis

Juliet E Compston and Clifford J Rosen
Sixth edition

www.fastfacts.com